Managing R
in Schizophrenia

MJ Travis • ER Peters • RW Kerwin

Institute of Psychiatry
London, UK

SCIENCE PRESS

Published by Science Press Ltd., 34–42 Cleveland Street, London W1T 4LB, UK.

http://current-science-group.com/

© 2001, Science Press Ltd.

British Library Cataloguing-in-Publication Data.

A catalogue record for this book is available from the British Library.

ISBN 1-85873-315-4

This book is supported by a grant from **AstraZeneca**. Sponsorship of this copy does not imply the sponsor's agreement with the opinions expressed herein.

Although every effort has been made to ensure that drug doses and other information are presented accurately in this publication, the ultimate responsibility rests with the prescribing physician. Neither the publishers nor the authors can be held responsible for errors or for any consequences arising from the use of the information contained herein. Any product mentioned in this publication should be used in accordance with the prescribing information prepared by the manufacturers. No claims or endorsements are made for any drug or compound at present under clinical investigation.

Editor: Sarah Findlay
Illustrator: Stuart Molloy
Designer: Claire Huntley
Typesetter: Simon Banister
Production controller: David Forrest

Printed in the UK.

Contents

Author biographies

Michael J Travis is a Lecturer in Clinical Neuropharmacology and Locum Consultant Psychiatrist at the Institute of Psychiatry and Maudsley Hospital, London, UK. He trained in medicine at Guy's Hospital and in psychiatry at St Bartholomew's and Hackney Hospitals, and The Royal Bethlem and Maudsley Hospitals, London, UK.

His main research interest is the study of drug action using functional imaging. Most recent contributions have been in the development of a novel ligand for the 5-HT$_{2A}$ receptor for single photon emission tomography and its use in clinical populations. Other clinical interests include clinical psychopharmacology and psychiatric intensive care. He has published several book chapters, in addition to original experimental research. Recent awards include a Young Investigator Award from the organisers of the International Congress on Schizophrenia Research 1999. Dr Travis is currently involved in setting up a pan-European collaborative study to probe the clinical relevance of neuro-receptor blockade in schizophrenia using single photon emission tomography.

Emmanuelle R Peters is a Lecturer in Clinical Psychology at the Institute of Psychiatry and Clinical Psychologist on the National Psychosis Unit, The Royal Bethlem Hospital and Maudsley Trust, London, UK. She trained in medicine at University College London, and received her PhD and clinical training at the Institute of Psychiatry, London, UK, followed by a Wellcome Post-Doctoral Fellowship.

After four years as a Lecturer at University College London, UK, she recently returned to the Institute of Psychiatry, London, UK, to pursue her clinical research interests in schizophrenia and cognitive-behaviour therapy for psychosis. She has taught under-graduate and medical students, psychiatrists, counsellors and clinical psychologists, and has published many articles in peer-reviewed journals in this field.

Robert W Kerwin is Professor of Clinical Neuropharmacology and Honorary Consultant Psychiatrist at the Institute of Psychiatry and Maudsley Hospital, London, UK, where he is head of a large research group. He is also Head of Clinical Pharmacology and Honorary Consultant Physician at King's College School of Medicine and Dentistry, London, UK. Professor Kerwin trained in medicine at Cambridge and Westminster Medical School, London, and in neuropharmacology at the University of Bristol, UK.

He is trained as a neuroreceptor pharmacologist and his main research interest is the study of antipsychotic drug action using functional imaging, pharmacogenetics and postmortem tissue. His most recent contributions have been in the elucidation of the mechanism of action of atypical drugs, development of the glutamate hypothesis of schizophrenia and development of allelic association studies in psychopharmacology. His other clinical interests include clinical psychopharmacology and psychiatric intensive care. Professor Kerwin has published four books, a wide range of reviews and chapters, and over 170 articles of original experimental research. Recent awards include a Doctor of the Year award for research merit, Hospital Team of the Year, jointly with Dr Reveley and Professor Murray, the Joel Elkes' International Award for outstanding contribution to neuropharmacology, and the SmithKlineBeecham Travelling Prize for outstanding contributions to clinical pharmacology.

Acknowledgements

Quotation on page 1. Wynne LC. **The natural histories of schizophrenic processes.** *Schizophr Bull* 1988; **14**:653–659.

Figure 1.1. Shepherd M, Watt D, Falloon I *et al.* **The natural history of schizophrenia: a five year follow-up study of outcome and prediction in a representative sample of schizophrenics.** *Psychol Med: Monogr Suppl* 1989; **15**:1–46.

Figure 1.2. Breier A, Schreiber JL, Dyer J *et al.* **National Institute of Mental Health longitudinal study of chronic schizophrenia.** *Arch Gen Psych* 1991; **48**:239–246. © 1991, American Medical Association.

Figure 1.3. Hegarty JD, Baldessarini RJ, Tohen H *et al.* **One hundred years of schizophrenia: a meta-analysis of the outcome literature.** *Am J Psychiatry* 1994; **151**:1409–1416.

Table 3.1. Schooler NR. **Maintenance medication for schizophrenia: Strategies for dose reduction.** *Schizophr Bull* 1991; **17**:311–324.

Figure 4.1. Schotte A, Janssen PF, Gommeren W *et al.* **Risperidone compared with new and reference antipsychotic drugs: in vitro and in vivo receptor binding.** *Psychopharmacol* (Berlin) 1996; **124**(1-2):57–73. © Springer-Verlag.

Table 4.2. Reprinted from Jibson MD, Tandon R. **New atypical antipsychotic medications.** *J Psychiatr Res* 1998; **32**(3/4):215–228. © 1998, with permission from Elsevier Science.

Table 5.4. Fowler D, Garety PA, Kuipers E. *Cognitive–Behaviour Therapy for Psychosis.* Chichester: John Wiley & Sons, Inc.; 1995. © John Wiley & Sons Limited. Reproduced with permission.

Table 5.5. Kemp R, David A, Hayward P. **Compliance therapy: An intervention targeting insight and treatment adherence in psychotic patients.** *Behav Cognitive Psychother* 1996; **24**:331–350.

Introduction

Schizophrenia is a heterogenous condition: the onset occurs during early adulthood and the illness commonly follows a chronic relapsing and remitting course. It is an inherently difficult illness to study because the definition of the schizophrenia syndrome varies with both time and location. This difficulty in assessment and definition affects all spheres of schizophrenia research, and consequently the results of outcome and natural history studies are influenced by factors such as differentiating course or outcome and the definition of remission and recovery. Similarly, treatment and intervention studies are affected by the choice of subject groups, the presence and type of control groups, and generalization of results to a clinical patient population.

The treatment of schizophrenia has been marked by three landmark events:

• the use of electroconvulsive therapy has been widespread since the 1930s, which has benefited some sufferers despite limited success in the treatment of schizophrenia and the prevention of relapse in general;
• arguably, the greatest advance was the discovery, and subsequent widespread use, of chlorpromazine and related antipsychotic medications. These medications are valuable in acute treatment and long-term prevention of relapse in schizophrenia. However, this generation of antipsychotics is far from ideal, producing quite marked, and potentially permanent, neurological side effects at therapeutic doses and providing little or no benefit to up to one-third of patients. This led to an understandable resistance to prescribing these medications for long-term use or early in the course of schizophrenia. Patient acceptability was also low, leading to high rates of noncompliance, or partial compliance, and an increased risk of relapse; and
• the re-introduction of clozapine and subsequent development of the 'atypical' or 'third generation' antipsychotics. Clozapine is the drug of choice for patients resistant to other antipsychotic medications and has an almost unique clinical profile. Other atypical antipsychotics shifted the clinical 'cost–benefit' ratio, with few side effects at therapeutic doses. These medications can, therefore, be used earlier in the course of illness and for longer periods, without the same concerns over long-term side effects.

We have attempted to briefly bring together selected evidence that illustrates the natural history of schizophrenia and the established benefits of older antipsychotics in the treatment of the illness. Advances in our understanding of the pharmacological management of schizophrenia are more fully discussed with reference to newer antipsychotics and their potential to improve the short-, medium- and long-term risk of relapse, and therefore the prognosis, of schizophrenia. There has been an increase in empirical research on evidence-based psychological therapy for psychosis, which has coincided with the renaissance of the pharmacotherapy of schizophrenia.

While medication remains the mainstay of treatment, it is becoming increasingly apparent that management and prevention of relapse in schizophrenia requires a combined, and evidence-based, pharmacological and psychological approach if the benefits of recent advances are to be translated into the general clinical setting.

Chapter 1

The natural history of schizophrenia

Introduction

"The natural history of an illness can be conceptualized as the untreated course of that illness — that is, as the trajectory that may be altered by treatment." [1; p. 653]

The importance of considering the natural history of schizophrenia lies at the heart of any assessment of treatment effectiveness, especially on the long-term outcome. As described in the Introduction, there are a number of methodological reasons that make the systematic and empirical evaluation of the natural history of schizophrenia problematic. Arguably, the most important confounder to any real knowledge of the natural history of schizophrenia is the fact that schizophrenia can seldom be allowed to follow a natural course, sufferers almost invariably require some kind of inter-vention in order to prevent harm or alleviate suffering. In addition, there is little data on subcategories of outcome before the introduction of neuroleptic therapy. Nevertheless, there is enough data to permit at least a preliminary insight.

Pre-somatic treatment (1895–1930)

Kraepelin initially considered dementia praecox to be an illness characterized by chronic deterioration. Similarly, Stearns [2] and Bleuler [3] stressed the negative therapeutic outcome in dementia praecox. However, in his own series of severe hos-pital-based cases, Kraepelin described a spontaneous and complete recovery in about 13–17% of patients [4]. In a meta-analysis, Hegarty *et al* [5] described that in 22 studies between 1895 and 1925, the average weighted proportion of patients diagnosed with Kraepelian dementia praecox that had a good outcome at follow up was in the region of 27.6%. Towards the end of this period the broader definition of dementia praecox as 'schizophrenia', stemming from Bleuler, became increasingly used and there was a corresponding improvement in the apparent outcome.

Pre-neuroleptic era (1930–1955)

During the pre-neuroleptic period there was increasing use of non-neuroleptic, somatic therapies, for example electroconvulsive therapy (ECT) and insulin. During this period, Hegarty *et al* [5] reported an improvement of approximately 35% in treat-ed men; however, much of this improvement would appear to be accounted for by the broadening of diagnostic criteria and, therefore, patients that may not have had schizophrenia, but rather an illness with a more favourable outcome, might have been included in the cohort.

It was toward the end of this period, and after the introduction of the first effective antipsychotic medications (neuroleptics), that studies combining rigorous reproducible diagnostic criteria and outcome measures were conducted. The IOWA 500 follow-up study probably provides the best insight into the natural history of schizophrenia [6]. In accordance with the available data between 1895 and 1925, of the 200 patients with schizophrenia meeting the narrow Feighner diagnostic criteria, only 26% of patients were discharged to the community following index hospitalization. These patients received institutional care as the only intervention. This figure is also similar to that determined by the Hegarty *et al* meta-analysis for patients diagnosed with schizophrenia by Kraepelian, non-Kraepelian and unspecified criteria, who received non-specific treatment and showed a good recovery across their study period [5].

Unfortunately, there is little stratified data on the 70–75% of patients in the preneuroleptic era who did not recover fully. Two large studies provide some information: Fuller [7], in a 15-year follow-up study (n = 1,200), reported that 25% of patients died during the study period, 35.3% were discharged from hospital at the end of the study, and 38.4% were chronically hospitalized throughout the study; and Malzburg [8], in a later study (n = 3,180), reported a much higher discharge rate in accordance with the move towards deinstitutionalization and the shorter follow-up period of three years. In this study, 59.3% of patients were discharged from hospital, 16.4% of the total cohort were classified as recovered, and 23.1% were much improved [9].

Post-neuroleptic era (1955–present)

The advent of neuroleptics as effective antipsychotics in the mid-1950s, and the introduction of clearer definitions of schizophrenia and outcome parameters has led to a much greater understanding of the potential outcomes of schizophrenia. Chapter 3 will consider whether the introduction of antipsychotic medication has altered the natural history of schizophrenia.

Hegarty *et al* [5] pooled data from 175 outcome studies in which patients received antipsychotic medication. They reported that across the groups in which either Kraepelian, non-Kraepelian, or unspecified criteria were used to diagnose schizophrenia roughly 45% of patients showed improvement. However, in the subsample of patients diagnosed using the narrower criteria only 31% improved.

One of the important advances in the literature on outcome has been the dozen or so studies that have prospectively followed up a group of patients with operationally defined schizophrenia over a number of years. A selection of these are presented in Table 1.1. The variability in outcome across these studies is clear and is due to a number of factors. The definition of schizophrenia varies between studies, as does the length of follow up and the criteria used to denote improvement. Moreover, the type of patient selected for follow up differs between studies, some are solely first-admission patients, some are chronic patients, and some of a mixture of the two. However, a useful breakdown of course types is provided by Shepherd *et al* [10]: the study followed up a cohort of patients with a present-state examination-defined diagnosis of schizophrenia that were admitted to a UK hospital over an 18-month period. Forty per cent of patients were first admissions. Of the initial cohort (n = 121), three had committed suicide, six had died of natural causes, and five were lost to follow up. The course of illness and outcome are illustrated in Figure 1.1.

Prospective studies of outcome in schizophrenia								
Study [reference]	No. of patients	Follow up (yrs)	Outcome or natural history of schizophrenia (%)					
			A	B	C	D	E	F
Stephens [11]	349	5–16	——— 24 ———			—— 46 ——		30
Alberta 2 [12]	43	14	21	30	12	–	21	16
Chestnut Lodge [13,14]	163	15	6	23	8	23	—— 41 ——	
Vermont Longitudinal Research Project [15]	82	32	–	45	17	—— 31 ——		7
Shepherd *et al* [10]	107	5	16	32	–	9	43	–
WHO collaborative study [16]	1352	2	38.9	21.1	–	–	–	39.8
Salokangas [17]	161	7.5–8	26.0	29	21*	–	–	24

* patients classified as having neurotic symptoms; A, recovered, one episode only – no impairment; B, periodic episodes, with no or minimal impairment; C, chronic mild impairment, without periodic exacerbations; D, periodic episodes, with chronic impairment after first episode; E, periodic episodes, with chronic impairment increasing after each episode; F, chronic severe impairment or psychotic symptoms, without periodic exacerbations. Please note that the figures in bold have been allocated to a specific category by the authors and that the original studies did not use the same outcome criteria as this table.

Table 1.1

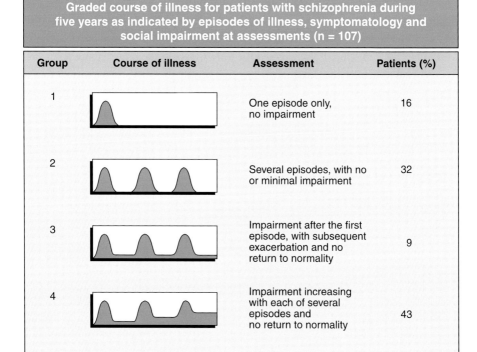

Group	Course of illness	Assessment	Patients (%)
1		One episode only, no impairment	16
2		Several episodes, with no or minimal impairment	32
3		Impairment after the first episode, with subsequent exacerbation and no return to normality	9
4		Impairment increasing with each of several episodes and no return to normality	43

Table title (spanning): Graded course of illness for patients with schizophrenia during five years as indicated by episodes of illness, symptomatology and social impairment at assessments (n = 107)

Figure 1.1. Adapted with permission from [10].

A common illness course?

Breier *et al* [18] (among others) have suggested that, despite the heterogeneity of schizophrenia, a model of a common course of illness can be derived. Based on evidence from their own studies and other long-term follow-up studies, the authors describe an early deteriorating phase, usually lasting about five years [19,20]. During this time there is a deterioration from pre-morbid levels of functioning that is often characterized by frank psychotic relapses. After this initial phase, much less fluctuation can be expected and the illness enters a 'stabilization' or 'plateau' phase [15,19]. This period may continue into the fifth decade when it is hypothesised that there is a third 'improving' phase for many patients (*see* Figure 1.2) [15,21].

Based on this type of model, it is tempting to suggest that adequate treatment interventions in the first five years will have a lasting effect on the course of a schizophrenic illness. This will be considered further in Chapter 2.

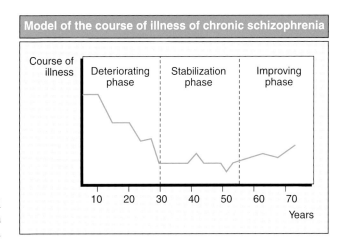

Figure 1.2. Adapted with permission from [18].

Conclusion

It is clear that there is a significant variation in the outcome and natural history of schizophrenia regardless of location, duration, or methods of the study. However, it would appear that schizophrenia is a chronic disease, frequently disabling for a lifetime, and with a worse outcome than other mental illnesses [20]. In addition, schizophrenia carries a high mortality. Rates of suicide in the studies quoted above and in Table 1.1 vary from about 2% to 10%, and overall the rate of suicide in schizophrenia is estimated to be in the region of between 10% and 13% [22,23].

In terms of treatment, there is considerable evidence that medication has a role in limiting the number and severity of relapses (*see* Chapter 3); however, the effect of medication on long-term outcome is less clear. Reviews of the literature related to the percentage of patients considered to be improved in follow-up studies of up to 10 years have failed to show any appreciable change in long-term outcome over the last 90 years (*see* Figure 1.3) [5,9]. Nevertheless, when these studies were analysed by treatment regimen the percentage of patients who showed improvement was significantly greater in cohorts treated with neuroleptic medication or convulsive therapy compared with other nonspecific methods or lobotomy, indicating a potential impact of medication on long-term outcome.

However, the fact that between 25% and 50% of patients fail to respond adequately to traditional antipsychotic medications [24] begs the exploration of improved treatments.

5

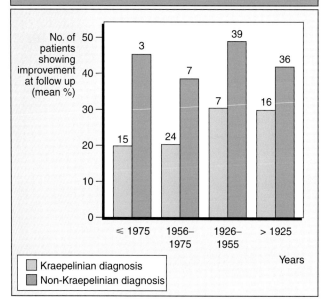

Mean percentages of schizophrenic patient cohorts considered improved in follow ups of at least 10 years

Figure 1.3. The numbers above each column indicate the number of cohorts for each era (total n = 147). The difference between outcomes across eras was highly significant with respect to diagnosis (p < 0.0001), with no significant effect of era or interaction and diagnosis. Adapted with permission from [5].

References

1. Wynne LC. **The natural histories of schizophrenic processes.** *Schizophr Bull* 1988; **14**(4):653–659.

2. Stearns AW. **The prognosis in dementia praecox.** *Boston Med Surg J* 1912; **167**:158–160.

3. Bleuler E. *Dementia Praecox or the group of schizophrenias.* New York: International Universities Press; 1911.

4. Kraepelin E. *Dementia Praecox and paraphrenia.* Translated by RM Barclay (1971). New York: Krieger Publishing Company; 1919.

5. Hegarty JD, Baldessarini RJ, Tohen H *et al.* **One hundred years of schizophrenia: a meta-analysis of the outcome literature.** *Am J Psychiatry* 1994; **151**:1409–1416.

6. Tsuang MT, Woolson RF, Fleming JA. **Long-term outcome of major psychoses I. Schizophrenia and affective disorders compared with psychiatrically symptom free surgical conditions.** *Arch Gen Psychiatry* 1979; **39**:1295–1301.

7. Fuller RG. **Hospital departures and readmissions among mental patients during the fifteen years following first admission.** *Psychiatr Q* 1930; **4**:642–689.

8. Malzberg B. **Rates of discharge and rates of mortality among first admissions to the New York Civil State Hospitals.** *Ment Hyg* 1952; **36**:619–638.

9. Van Os J, Wright P, Murray RM. **Follow-up studies of schizophrenia I: natural history and non-psychopathological predictors of outcome.** *Eur Psychiatry* 1997; **12**(suppl. 5):327s–341s.

10. Shepherd M, Watt D, Falloon I *et al*. **The natural history of schizophrenia: a five year follow-up study of outcome and prediction in a representative sample of schizophrenics.** *Psychol Med: Monogr Suppl* 1989; **15**:1–46.

11. Stephens JH. **Long-term course and prognosis in schizophrenia.** *Sem Psychiatry* 1970; **2**:464–485.

12. Bland RC, Orn H. **Fourteen year outcome in early schizophrenia.** *Acta Psychiatrica Scand* 1978; **58**:327–338.

13. McGlashan TH. **The Chestnut Lodge follow-up study: I. Follow-up methodology and study sample.** *Arch Gen Psychiatry* 1984; **41**:573–585.

14. McGlashan TH. **The Chestnut Lodge follow-up study:II. Long term outcome of schizophrenia and the affective disorders.** *Arch Gen Psychiatry* 1984; **41**:586–601.

15. Harding CM, Brooks GW, Ashikaga T *et al*. **The Vermont Longitudinal study of persons with severe metal illness: II. Long term outcome of subjects who retrospectively met DSM-III criteria for schizophrenia.** *Am J Psychiatry* 1987; **144**:727–735.

16. Sartorius N, Jablensky A, Korten A *et al*. **Early manifestations and first contact incidence of schizophrenia in different cultures.** *Psychol Med* 1986; **16**:909–928.

17. Salokangas RKR. **Prognostic implications of the sex of schizophrenic patients.** *Br J Psychiatry* 1983; **142**:145–151.

18. Breier A, Schreiber JL, Dyer J *et al*. **National Institute of Mental Health Longitudinal Study of Chronic Schizophrenia.** *Arch Gen Psych* 1991; **48**:239–246.

19. Carpenter WT, Strauss JS. **The prediction of outcome in schizophrenia. IV: Eleven year follow-up of the Washington IPSS cohort.** *J Nerv Ment Dis* 1991; **179**:517–525.

20. McGlashan TH. **A selective review of recent North American Long-Term Follow-up Studies of Schizophrenia.** *Schizophr Bull* 1988; **14**(4):515–542.

21. Bleuler M. *The schizophrenic disorders: Long Term Patient and Family studies.* New Haven: Yale University Press; 1978.

22. Caldwell CB, Gottesman II. **Schizophrenics kill themselves too: a review of risk factors for suicide.** *Schizophr Bull* 1990; **16**:571–589.

23. Roy A. **Suicide in Chronic Schizophrenia.** *Br J Psychiatry* 1982; **141**:171–177.

24. Kane J, Honigfeld G, Singer J *et al*. **Clozapine for the treatment-resistant schizophrenic: double blind comparison with chlorpromazine.** *Arch Gen Psychiatry* 1988; **45**:789–796.

Chapter 2

Prognosis in schizophrenia

Introduction

Factors traditionally thought to predict poor prognosis are listed in Table 2.1. Although all of the factors in this list have been firmly associated with poorer outcome [1], most account for less than 10% in variance, with only duration of symptoms prior to treatment accounting for up to 20% of the variance of outcome [2]. The evidence for some of these predictors will be considered in this Chapter.

Factors linked with a poor prognosis in schizophrenia
Early onset
Insidious onset
Poor premorbid personality
Long period between onset of symptoms and treatment
Male sex
Lack of prominent affective component
Lack of clear precipitants
Family history of schizophrenia
Low IQ
Low social class
Social isolation
Previous psychiatric history

Table 2.1. IQ, intelligence quotient.

Age and type of onset

It has been frequently reported that an earlier age at onset, usually less than 20 years old, and an insidious — as opposed to acute onset of illness — predict a poorer prognosis for patients with schizophrenia [3–6]. Given that poor premorbid functioning is associated with poor outcome it makes intuitive sense that an individual will be impaired to a larger extent if onset of illness occurs during the phase of emotional maturation.

Premorbid functioning

The findings outlined above correspond with the association between an earlier age of onset and poorer performance prior to the onset of symptoms seen both occupationally and academically in patients with schizophrenia compared with their peers

9

[5]. Indeed, good premorbid functioning has been consistently associated with a better outcome, particularly in the first ten years following index discharge [7,8].

Effect of length of illness prior to treatment

The evidence that a longer duration of illness prior to treatment is detrimental to various measures of treatment outcome is based on a number of retrospective analyses and three prospective studies.

Effect of the introduction of neuroleptic therapy on outcome

Wyatt [9] reviewed a series of 19 studies, of primarily first-onset patients, which compared the outcome of those treated before the advent of chlorpromazine with those treated subsequently. He noted that the use of medication increased the chance of better long-term course. This conclusion was supported by Opjordsmoen [10], who compared first-time admission of patients with delusional states (n = 151), half of whom were admitted prior to neuroleptic treatment and half afterwards. Despite the fact that all of Opjordsmoen's cohort received neuroleptics at some point in the course of their illness, the author described a significantly worse outcome for the patients that did not receive neuroleptics as their first treatment.

Retrospective studies

In a review of 10 studies relating to the first wave of patients treated with neuroleptics, Angrist and Schulz [11] reported than in six out of ten patients the response to pharmacotherapy correlated negatively with duration of illness. Results supporting these findings have been noted in studies from China [12], Japan [13], and Iceland [14]. The latter study split their group (n = 107) on the basis of pretreatment illness of greater than or less than one year. They reported that during 18-years follow up the group with pretreatment illness greater than one year had a higher readmission rate. A smaller but significant study (n = 20), demonstrated that the ongoing treatment for patients with greater than six-months pretreatment illness cost twice as much as ongoing treatment for those who received treatment within six months of the onset of symptoms over a follow-up period of three years [15].

Prospective studies

Three major prospective studies focusing on the duration of pretreatment illness have found an association between longer duration of illness and poorer outcome.

In the smaller study reporting this association, Rabiner *et al* [16] investigated a sample of 36 first-episode psychotic patients over one year and reported a correlation between relapse or poor outcome and longer duration of pretreatment illness in the group with schizophrenia. In a larger study, Johnstone *et al* [17] reported on a sample of 253 first onset patients with schizophrenia followed up for two years. In this sample, patients with a longer duration of illness had a higher frequency of relapse. This effect was observed in patients included in both placebo or active treatment groups of the controlled trial, emphasising the importance of early treatment [18].

In a widely quoted two-year follow-up study, Loebel *et al* [19] used an antipsychotic treatment protocol to carefully and intensively investigate 70 first-episode patients diagnosed with either schizophrenia or schizoaffective disorder: the majority of patients in this study had schizophrenia. The authors separated duration of illness prior to treatment into two components, the first included the duration of the prodrome plus the duration of psychotic symptoms, and the second duration of psychotic symptoms alone. The study reported that a lower level of remission was associated with a longer duration of both psychotic symptoms and prodrome prior to treatment. Increased duration of pretreatment psychotic symptoms was associated with increased time to remission. Importantly, time to remission was not related to other factors, although a lower level of remission was associated with poorer premorbid functioning and an earlier age at onset. This finding of an association between better treatment response and shorter duration of pretreatment psychosis has recently been replicated by Szymanski *et al* [20].

Sex

It is generally thought that women with schizophrenia have a better prognosis than men. Certainly, in samples drawn from first- and recent-onset cases women appear to spend less time in psychosis, are readmitted to hospital less frequently, have less social impairment, live independently more often, and spend more time in remission [6,21–25]. Men appear to be almost twice as likely as women to have at least mild social impairment at follow up and half as likely to experience complete remission [23,26].

This sex difference is not as evident in samples drawn from chronic populations, possibly reflecting the exclusion of women with a favourable outcome or an attenuation of the sex differences in outcome [26].

The reasons for this sex difference are unclear. Although some of the variation can be explained by differences in age of onset, marital status, and premorbid adjustment, a further problem is the difference in the expression of the illness in women who are more likely to present with affective symptoms that are associated with a better outcome.

11

Symptom type

Variations in long-term outcome and prognosis in schizophrenia has been associated with a variety of different symptom clusters. Fenton and McGlashan [27] describe a better outcome for paranoid versus nonparanoid patients, but also a later age of onset. They also reported an association between schizophrenia with prominent negative symptoms at onset and partial or no remission in the first few years of illness [28]. In particular, prominent negative symptoms were associated with other predictors of poor outcome, for example poor premorbid functioning and insidious onset of symptoms. The presence of strong affective features at onset of illness is associated with a better prognosis [7,29]. This is mirrored in results showing that patients with a diagnosis of schizoaffective disorder have a relatively better outcome compared with patients suffering from 'pure' schizophrenia [1,30].

Substance misuse

The relationship between substance misuse and schizophrenia is complex. Many drugs of abuse (eg, ketamine, amphetamine and lysergic diethylamide) are psychotomimetic, and care must be taken to avoid the misdiagnosis of a drug-induced psychosis as schizophrenia. Psychoactive substance misuse both preceeds and follows the onset of psychotic symptoms. Substantiation that subgroups of patients receive transient symptom reduction from some abused drugs further complicates this picture, and it may well be that some patients are 'self-medicating' with drugs of abuse [31].

It is estimated that between 20% and 47% of the population with schizophrenia may qualify as dual-diagnosis patients [32,33]. Such patients have a higher use of services and a worse outcome than patients that are not abusers [34]. Swofford *et al* [35] reported that during an antipsychotic dose-reduction study substance abusers were twice as likely to be hospitalized and had four times as many relapses as the non-user group during the two-year follow-up period. It is interesting to note that patients with schizophrenia seem to suffer significant harm at lower levels of substance use [36]. In a recent study of substance misuse in schizophrenic patients in Camberwell (London, UK), 20.5% of the dual-diagnosis patients had alcohol problems only, 4.7% had drug problems only, and 11.1% had drug and alcohol problems. In this sample, men were between two and three times more likely to abuse substances than women, there was no observed difference between white and black patients. All the dual-diagnosis patients had increased lengths of admission to hospital [37].

As substance misuse is so prevalent, this is an area where secondary prevention of relapse could be focused.

Family history

Family studies have indicated that a history of schizophrenia is associated with increased 'genetic loading' or propensity to develop schizophrenia [38]. Some studies have indicated that genetic loading is greater among patients with the poor-prognosis nonparanoid subtypes of schizophrenia without firm evidence that subtypes 'breed-true' [39,40]. Therefore, there is probably a link between a family history of schizophrenia per se and a poorer outcome.

Psychosocial factors

Generally, most of the studies quoted in this Chapter have indicated that poor psychosocial functioning, on the various parameters used in each study, is associated with poor outcome. These parameters include social isolation and low social class. Increasing social isolation is often part of the prodromal phase of a schizophreniform illness, however, several studies have associated a premorbid schizoid personality or a tendency to be a 'loner' with a poor outcome at follow up [41–43].

There appears to be a relationship between low social class and poor outcome in the first 2–5 years of illness. Studies in the UK [44,45] and the US [46] have consistently shown that with a decrease in social class there is an increasing likelihood of patients having an unremitting poorly treatment-responsive illness and remaining in hospital. There is also a decreased likelihood of lower social class patients gaining benefit from rehabilitation.

The psychosocial aspects of relapse prevention will be considered in Chapter 5.

Conclusion

Despite a number of firm associations between various factors and outcome in schizophrenia their predictive value and potential for use in the clinical setting is limited. One of the possible benefits of the data on length of illness prior to treatment is to inform strategies for intervention in order to limit poor prognosis. Strategies to identify individuals who are at high risk of developing psychosis and provide early intervention are the subject of intense research but are time consuming and costly. Nevertheless patients with a confirmed first episode of psychosis are a group where effective early intervention with appropriate medications may reap medium and long-term gains in terms of improved prognosis and subsequent decreased risk of relapse.

References

1. World Health Organisation. *Schizophrenia: An International Follow-up study.* Chichester: John Wiley & Sons, Inc.; 1979.

2. Moller HJ, Von Zerssen D. **Course and outcome of schizophrenia.** In: *Schizophrenia.* Edited by SR Hirsch and DR Weinberger. Oxford: Blackwell Science Ltd.; 1995, 106–127.

3. Stephens JH. **Long-term course and prognosis in schizophrenia.** *Sem Psychiatry* 1970; **2**:464–485.

4. Stoffelmayer BE, Dillavou D, Hunter JE. **Premorbid functioning and outcome in schizophrenia: a cumulative analysis.** *J Consult Clin Psychol* 1983; **51**:338–352.

5. Johnstone EC, MacMillan JF, Frith CD *et al.* **Further investigation of the predictors of outcome following first schizophrenic episodes.** *Br J Psychiatry* 1990; **157**:182–189.

6. Jablensky A, Sartorius N, Ernberg G *et al.* **Schizophrenia: manifestations, incidence and course in different cultures. A WHO ten country study.** *Psychol Med Monogr Suppl* 1992; **20**:1–97.

7. Stephens JH. **Long-term prognosis and follow up in schizophrenia.** *Schizophr Bull* 1978; **4**:25–47.

8. McGlashan TH. **Predictors of shorter-, medium-, and longer-term outcome in schizophrenia.** *Am J Psychiatry* 1986; **143**:50–55.

9. Wyatt RJ. **Neuroleptics and the natural course of schizophrenia.** *Schizophr Bull* 1991; **17**:325–351.

10. Opjordsmoen S. **Long-term clinical outcome of schizophrenia with special reference to gender differences.** *Acta Psychiatr Scand* 1991; **83**:307–313.

11. Angrist B, Shulz SC. *Introduction to the Neuroleptic Non-responsive Patient: Characterization and Treatment.* Washington: American Psychiatric Press; 1990.

12. Lo WH, Lo T. **A ten-year follow-up study of Chinese schizophrenics in Hong Kong.** *Br J Psychiatry* 1977; **131**:63–66.

13. Inoue K, Nakajima T, Kato N. **A longitudinal study of schizophrenia in adolescence: I the one to three year outcome.** *Jpn J Psychiatry Neurol (Tokyo)* 1986; **40**:143–151.

14. Helgason L. **Twenty years' follow-up of first psychiatric presentation for schizophrenia: What could have been prevented.** *Acta Psychiatr Scand* 1990; **81**:231–235.

15. Moscarelli M, Capri S, Neri L. **Cost evaluation of chronic schizophrenic patients during the first three years after first contact.** *Schizophr Bull* 1991; **17**(3):421–426.

16. Rabiner CJ, Wegner JT, Kane JM. **Outcome study of first episode psychosis: Relapse rates after 1 year.** *Am J Psychiatry* 1986; **143**(9):1155–1158.

17. Johnstone EC, Crow TJ, Johnson AL *et al.* **The Northwick Park Study of first episode schizophrenia: Presentation of the illness and problems relating to admission.** *Br J Psychiatry* 1986; **148**:115–120.

18. Crow TJ, MacMillan JF, Johnson AL *et al.* **A randomised controlled trial of prophylactic neuroleptic treatment.** *Br J Psychiatry* 1986; **148**:120–127.

19. Loebel AD, Lieberman JA, Alvir JM *et al.* **Duration of Psychosis and Outcome in First-Episode Schizophrenia.** *Am J Psychiatry* 1992; **149**(9):1183–1188.

20. Szymanski SR, Cannon TD, Gallacher F *et al.* **Course and treatment response in first episode and chronic schizophrenia.** *Am J Psychiatry* 1996; **153**: 519–525.

21. Salokangas RKR. **Prognostic implications of the sex of schizophrenic patients.** *Br J Psychiatry* 1983; **142**: 145–151.

22. Goldstein JM. **Sex differences in the course of schizophrenia.** *Am J Psychiatry* 1988; **145**: 684–689.

23. Shepherd M, Watt D, Falloon I et al. **The natural history of schizophrenia: a five year follow-up study of outcome and prediction in a representative sample of schizophrenics.** *Psychol Med Monogr Suppl* 1989; **15**:1–46.

24. Angermeyer MC, Kuhn L, Goldstein JM. **Gender and the course of schizophrenia: differences in treated outcomes.** *Schizophr Bull* 1990; **16**:293–307.

25. Navarro F, van Os J, Jones P et al. **Explaining sex differences in outcome in functional psychoses.** *Schizophr Res* 1996; **21**:161–170.

26. Van Os J, Wright P Murray R. **Follow-up studies of schizophrenia I: natural history and non-psychopathological predictors of outcome.** *European Psychiatry* 1997; **12**(suppl. 5): 327s–341s.

27. Fenton WS, McGlashan TH. **Natural History of schizophrenia subtypes: I. Longitudinal study of paranoid, hebephrenic and undifferentiated schizophrenia.** *Arch Gen Psychiatry* 1991; **144**:1306–1309.

28. Fenton WS, McGlashan TH. **Natural history of schizophrenia subtypes: II. Positive and negative symptoms and long term course.** *Arch Gen Psychiatry* 1991; **48**:978–986.

29. Fenton WS, McGlashan TH. **Sustained remission in drug-free schizophrenics.** *Am J Psychiatry* 1987; **144**:969–977.

30. Tsuang MT, Woolson RF, Fleming JA. **Long-term outcome of major psychoses I. Schizophrenia and affective disorders compared with psychiatrically symptom free surgical conditions.** *Arch Gen Psychiatry* 1979; **36**(12): 1295–1301.

31. Dixon L, Haas G, Weiden PJ et al. **Drug abuse in schizophrenic patients: clinical correlates and reasons for use.** *Am J Psychiatry* 1991; **148**(2): 224–230.

32. Barbee JG, Clark PD, Crapanzano MS et al. **Alcohol and substance abuse among schizophrenic patients presenting to an emergency psychiatric service.** *J Nerv Ment Dis* 1989; **177**(7): 400–407.

33. Regier DA, Farmer ME, Rae DS et al. **Comorbidity of mental disorders with alcohol and other drug abuse. Results from the Epidemiologic Catchment Area (ECA) Study [see comments].** *JAMA* 1990; **264**(19):2511–2518.

34. Lehman AF, Myers CP, Thompson JW et al. **Implications of mental and substance use disorders. A comparison of single and dual diagnosis patients.** *J Nerv Ment Dis* 1993; **181**(6):365–370.

35. Swofford CD, Kasckow JW, Scheller-Gilkey G et al. **Substance use: a powerful predictor of relapse in schizophrenia.** *Schizophr Res* 1996; **20**(1–2):145–151.

36. Drake RE, Wallach MA. **Moderate drinking among people with severe mental illness.** *Hosp Community Psychiatry* 1993; **44**(8):780–782.

37. Menezes PR, Johnson S, Thornicroft G *et al.* **Drug and alcohol problems among individuals with severe mental illness in south London.** *Br J Psychiatry* 1996; **168**:612–619.

38. Kendler KS, Davis KL. **The genetics and biochemistry of paranoid schizophrenia and other paranoid psychoses.** *Schizophr Bull* 1981; **7**:689–709.

39. Jorgensen A, Teasdale TW, Parnas J *et al.* **The Copenhagen high-risk project. The diagnosis of maternal schizophrenia and its relation to offspring diagnosis.** *Br J Psychiatry* 1987; **151**:753–757.

40. McGuffin P, Farmer AE, Gottesman II *et al.* **Twin concordance for operationally defined schizophrenia. Confirmation of familiality and hereditability.** *Arch Gen Psychiatry* 1984; **41**(6):541–545.

41. Bland RC and Orn H. **Prediction of long-term outcome from presenting symptoms in schizophrenia.** *J Clin Psychiatry* 1980; **41**:85–88.

42. Stephens JH, Astrup C, Carpenter WT *et al.* **A comparison of nine systems to diagnose schizophrenia.** *Psychiatry Res* 1982; **6**:127–143.

43. Tsuang MT, Woolson RF, Winokur G *et al.* **Stability of psychiatric diagnosis: Schizophrenia and affective disorders followed up over a 30 to 40 year period.** *Arch Gen Psychiatry* 1981; **38**:535–539.

44. Cooper JE. **Social Class and Prognosis in Schizophrenia.** *British Journal of Prevent Soc Med* 1961; **15**:17–41.

45. McKenzie K, van Os J, Fahy T *et al.* **Evidence for good prognosis psychosis among UK Afro-Caribbeans.** *Br Med J* 1995; **311**:1325–1328.

46. Myers JK, Bean LL. *A decade later: a follow up of social class and mental illness.* Chichester: John Wiley & Sons, Inc.; 1968.

Chapter 3

Pharmacotherapy for acute schizophrenia

Introduction

The fortuitous discovery of chlorpromazine in the early 1950s heralded an era of effective pharmacological treatment for schizophrenia. Since the initial 1952 report of reduced agitation, aggression and delusional states in schizophrenic patients treated with chlorpromazine there have been a wealth of placebo-controlled trials establishing the efficacy of neuroleptic antipsychotic medication for acute schizophrenia. The best-known large-scale clinical trial, which gives a good idea of the effect size to be expected, was carried out by The National Institute of Mental Health, USA [1]. This study involved four treatment groups, (chlorpromazine, thioridazine, fluphenazine, and placebo) with 90 randomly allocated subjects in each. The subjects were treated for six weeks and rated on 14 different symptoms, in addition to global clinical improvement. In this study, 75% of individuals in the chlorpromazine-, thioridazine- and fluphenazine-treated groups showed significant improvement, 5% failed to be helped, and 2% deteriorated. Only 25% of individuals in the placebo group showed significant improvements, and over 50% were unchanged or worse. A reanalysis of these results indicated that improvement occurred across all 14 symptom areas, including both positive and negative symptoms [2], although there was no difference between the active drugs.

Davis and Andriukaitis [3] performed a meta-analysis using the trials involving chlorpromazine, investigated the relationship between dose and clinical effect. They noted that a threshold dose of 400 mg of chlorpromazine is required based on the meta-analysis of 31 trials using a dose of at least 400 mg of chlorpromazine per day; only one trial had failed to show that chlorpromazine was less effective than the reference treatment. In the 31 trials using a dose less than 400 mg of chlorpromazine, 19 had failed to show a significant improvement over reference treatment.

Pharmacotherapy as a maintenance treatment in schizophrenia

Although it is widely accepted that antipsychotic medication is the mainstay of treatment in acute schizophrenia its role in long-term maintenance has been more contentious. Nevertheless, the importance of maintenance drug therapy in the treatment of chronic schizophrenia has been evident since the early 1960s.

Initial studies indicated that between half and two-thirds of patients with schizophrenia who were stabilized on medication relapsed following cessation of maintenance pharmacological therapy compared with between 5% and 30% of patients maintained on medication [4–6]. Two recent reviews have collated the information from trials in which antipsychotics were withdrawn from populations of patients with schizophrenia that had responded to medication [7,8].

In a review of 66 studies between 1958 and 1993, Gilbert *et al* [7] noted that relapse rates in the medication withdrawal groups was 53.2% (follow-up period of between 6.3 and 9.7 months) compared with 15.6% (follow-up period of 7.9 months) in the maintenance group. There was also a positive relationship between risk of relapse and length of follow up. Viguera *et al* [8] used data from 22 patient cohorts, and investigated the relationship between gradual (last depot injection or tailing off over at least three weeks) and abrupt medication discontinuation. They noted a cumulative relapse rate of about 46% at six-month follow up, and 56.2% at 24-month follow up in patients whose medication was stopped abruptly. They calculated that in patients whose medication was stopped gradually the relapse rate at six months was halved. They also described that 50% of inpatients had relapsed by five months after cessation of medication while in the outpatient group relapse rates remained less than 50% after four-year follow up.

Therefore, findings from medication discontinuation studies have conclusively shown, as a group, patients with schizophrenia fare better if they receive antipsychotic medication. However, prolonged use of antipsychotic medication, particularly the older typical antipsychotics, carries a high risk of adverse effects, especially tardive dyskinesia. In order to attempt to minimize the risk of these events, much recent work has focused on the use of low-dose medication regimens and intermittent dosing strategies and atypical drug therapy.

Low-dose antipsychotics

The rationale underlying the use of low-dose strategies is that significantly lower doses of medication are required for maintenance, as opposed to the acute, treatment of schizophrenia. This assumes that all major treatment goals have been met for the patients by the time of dose reduction. The two major aims are to ensure that the stability of symptomatic improvement is at least maintained, and to minimize the risk of neurological side effects and secondary negative symptoms caused by higher doses of typical antipsychotics.

A number of trials have investigated the use of standard doses of depot antipsychotics (between 250 and 500 mg chlorpromazine equivalents) in comparison with continuous 'low-dose' regimens, usually at least 50% less [9,10]. On the whole, these studies have indicated that the patients treated with lower doses of antipsychotics have a higher rate of exacerbation of their psychotic symptoms and higher rates of relapse.

Using the results of six selected studies, Barbui *et al* [10] quote a relative risk of relapse of between 45% and 65% in the lowest-dose group at 12-month follow up, with the relapse rate highest in the low-dose group (50 mg chlorpromazine equivalents per day). Most of the studies did, however, report a lower incidence of extrapyramidal side effects and fewer symptoms of anxiety or negative symptoms [9]. There are a number of limitations to these studies, not least that the doses used in the standard groups are in the low-to-moderate dose range. Also, no systematic evaluation has been carried out of the patient characteristics likely to predict a good response to lower dose therapy.

Intermittent or targeted medication

This treatment strategy is based on the assumption that patients can be maintained on intermittently administered low doses of antipsychotics. There are two strategies: (i) the patient only takes medication for four days of the week, having a 'drug holiday' for the other three days [11]. Although this strategy does not seem to increase relapse rates, patients still developed tardive dyskinesia. (ii) Targeted treatment has been the subject of systematic research and is based on the assumption that patients only require antipsychotic medication while symptomatic. The rationale is that if the patient's total 'medication load' can be reduced then rates of tardive dyskinesia will be lower and social functioning may be improved. Targeted treatment relies on a close collaboration between patients and carers, and the identification of a signature 'prodrome' that warns of an incipient relapse. During prodrome medication can be given to the patient and a full relapse avoided.

Table 3.1 shows the results from four trials of targeted treatment. In the Herz *et al* [12] and Carpenter *et al* [13] studies patients were seen on a weekly basis, either in the form of supportive group therapy and family education or on a one-to-one basis. If prodromal signs were noted a known medication was substituted for placebo and administered until the patient was re-stabilized. In both studies, the targeted groups received less total medication, but had more frequent prodromal signs and relapses. However, rehospitalization and psychopathology did not differ between the two groups at two-year follow up. In the Jolley *et al* study [14], patients were seen every four weeks and the families received a one-hour teaching session. At one year the results mirrored those outlined above, and side effects were less in the targeted group. However, at two years the targeted groups, while still receiving less total medication, had a higher rate of relapse and hospitalization. Gaebel *et al* [15] have reported on a cohort of 365 patients, using a similar design to that described above. They included a group of patients who only received medication when 'in crisis' rather than at the identification of prodromal symptoms. This 'crisis' group did significantly less well than the early intervention group, with three times as many relapsing within the first six months. The two-year analysis of both continuous medication and targeted groups

Maintenance targeted or intermittent treatment studies				
Study characteristics	Herz et al [12]	Carpenter et al [13]	Jolley et al [14]	Gaebel et al [15]
n	101	116	54	365
Patient population	Outpatients	Recently discharged	Outpatients	Recently hospitalized
Stabilization	3 months	8 weeks	6 months	3 months postdischarge
Psychosocial support	Weekly support groups	Individual case managers	Monthly RN/MD visits	Special outpatient clinics
Control features	Random/ double blind	Random/ double blind	Random/FLU decanoate double blind	Random/ nonblind
Study Results				
Dosage: continued targeted early targeted crisis	290^3 150	1.7^2 1.0	$1,616^4$ 298	208 91 118^5
12 month relapse (%): continued targeted early	10 29	33 55	9 22	15 35
24 month relapse (%): continued targeted early	17 36	39 62	14 54	23 49
[1] Treatment was for 24 months in all studies; [2] 1 = low (eg, less than 30 mg chlorpromazine) and 2 = moderate (eg, 301–600 mg/day); [3] mg/day expressed in chlorpromazine equivalents; [4] mean total dose expressed in haloperidol equivalents; [5] cumulative dosage over two years in (1,000 g) chlorpromazine.				

Table 3.1. FLU, fluphenazine; MD, physician; RN, registered nurse. Adapted with permission from [16].

indicated that there were significantly more relapses and more frequent hospitalizations (37% versus 24%, respectively) in the early intervention group compared with patients receiving continuous medication. However, employment rates in the two groups were similar (approximately 50%).

Therefore, in summary it appears that patients receiving intermittent targeted therapy while receiving less medication than those on continuous therapy have a higher rate of relapse and may have a higher rate of re-hospitalization. At two years, however, there is little difference in social functioning or psychopathology between the two groups.

Conclusion

Despite overwhelming evidence that antipsychotic medication is the most effective strategy in preventing relapse in schizophrenia there is still considerable scope for improvement. A wealth of research has been directed at the optimal use of older antipsychotics, yet there is no clear consensus on the best dose–frequency–duration strategy required to provide a comfortable balance between the risk of unwanted side effects and the aim of protecting against relapse. The reintroduction of clozapine and the development of 'atypical' antipsychotics, with their more favourable side effect profile, has produced a good degree of optimism that some of the more pervading problems of relapse prevention in schizophrenia may have a solution.

References

1. NIMH Psychopharmacology Service Centre Study Group. **Phenothiazine treatment in schizophrenia.** *Arch Gen Psychiatry* 1964; **10**:246–226.

2. Goldberg SC, Klerman GL, Cole JO *et al.* **Changes in Schizophrenic psychopathology and ward behaviour as a function of phenthiazine treatment.** *Br J Psychiatry* 1965; **111**:120–133.

3. Davis JM, Andriukaitis S. **The natural course of schizophrenia and effective maintenance treatment.** *J Clin Psychopharmacol* 1986; **6**(suppl.):2–10.

4. Caffey EM, Diamond LS, Frank TV *et al.* **Discontinuation or reduction of chemotherapy in chronic schizophrenics.** *J Chronic Dis* 1964; **17**:347–358.

5. Hogarty GE, Goldberg SC, Schooler NR *et al.* **Drug and sociotherapy in the aftercare of schizophrenic patients. II: two year relapse rates.** *Arch Gen Psychiatry* 1974; **31**:603–608.

6. Davis JM. **Overview:maintenance therapy in psychiatry. I: Schizophrenia.** *Am J Psychiatry* 1975; **132**:1237–1245.

7. Gilbert PL, Harris J, McAdams LA *et al.* **Neuroleptic withdrawal in schizophrenic patients.** *Arch Gen Psychiatry* 1995; **52**:173–188.

8. Viguera AC, Baldessarini RJ, Hegarty JD *et al.* **Clinical risk following abrupt and gradual withdrawal of maintenance neuroleptic treatment.** *Arch Gen Psychiatry* 1997; **54**:49–55.

9. Schooler NA. **Reducing dosage in maintenance treatment of schizophrenia.** *Br J Psychiatry* 1993; **163**(suppl. 22):58–65.

10. Barbui C, Saraceno B, Liberati A *et al*. **Low-dose neuroleptic therapy and relapse in schizophrenia: meta-analysis of randomized controlled trials.** *European Psychiatry* 1996; **11**:306–313.

11. McCreadie RG, Dingwall JM, Wiles DH *et al*. **Intermittent pimozide versus fluphenazine decanoate as maintenance therapy in chronic schizophrenia.** *Br J Psychiatry* 1980; **137**:510–517.

12. Herz MI, Glazer WM, Mostert MA *et al*. **Intermittent vs maintenance medication in schizophrenia. Two-year results.** *Arch Gen Psychiatry* 1991; **48**(4):333–339.

13. Carpenter WT Jr., Hanlon TE, Heinrichs DW *et al*. **Continuous versus targeted medication in schizophrenic outpatients: outcome results [published erratum appears in Am J Psychiatry 1991 Jun;148(6):819].** *Am J Psychiatry* 1990; **147**(9):1138–1148.

14. Jolley AG, Hirsch SR, Morrison E *et al*. **Trial of brief intermittent neuroleptic prophylaxis for selected schizophrenic outpatients: clinical and social outcome at two years.** *Br Med J* 1990; **301**:837–842.

15. Gaebel W, Frick U, Köpcke W *et al*. **Early neuroleptic intervention in schizophrenia: are prodromal symptoms valid predictors of relapse?** *Br J Psychiatry Suppl* 1993; **163**(21):8–12.

16. Schooler NR. **Maintenance medication for schizophrenia: Strategies for dose reduction.** *Schizophr Bull* 1991; **17**:311–324.

Chapter 4

Are new antipsychotics superior maintenance treatments?

Introduction

The reintroduction of clozapine in 1990 and the advent of several new antipsychotics over the past few years has renewed interest and optimism in the treatment of schizophrenia. These newer antipsychotics have, for want of a better term, been classified as 'atypical antipsychotics'. This term has a variety of definitions, tells us little about the pharmacology of the drug, and does not aid the clinician in prescribing. A new classification is outlined in Table 4.1. The new 'atypical antipsychotics' are better called 'third generation antipsychotics'. The rationale for this is that the first generation antipsychotics were developed from the known pharmacology and structure of chlorpromazine and share high dopamine D_2 receptor occupancy as their primary mode of action. Second generation antipsychotics include drugs such as sulpiride, thioridazine, and remoxipride. Using current definitions these may be classified as 'atypical antipsychotics'. They still appear to exert their effects via D_2 receptor antagonism, but do not seem to confer the benefits of the third generation drugs. The third generation of antipsychotics has been developed using clozapine, rather than chlorpromazine, as a prototype. Although drugs of this class have a variable pharmacology they may exert their effects via other receptors, for example the serotonin (5-hydroxytryptamine [5-HT])$_{2A}$ receptor,

Classification of antipsychotics agents
First generation antipsychotics (otherwise known as 'typical' antipsychotics)
Based on the structure and pharmacology of chlorpromazine (ie, chlorpromazine, haloperidol, zuclopenthixol, stelazine)
Second generation antipsychotics
Next stage in drug development, may be 'atypical' by some definitions (ie, sulpiride, remoxipride, thioridazine)
Third generation antipsychotics (otherwise known as 'atypical' antipsychotics)
Based on the structure and/or pharmacology of clozapine:

Broad spectrum	*Serotonin/dopamine antagonist*
clozapine	risperidone
olanzapine	sertindole
quetiapine	ziprasidone

Table 4.1

in addition to the D_2 receptor. The third generation drugs may be subdivided further on the basis of their relative affinities for a range of receptors into 'broad-spectrum third generation' (eg, clozapine, olanzapine and quetiapine) and 'serotonin–dopamine antagonist (SDA) third generation' (eg, risperidone, sertindole and ziprasidone). Figure 4.1 shows that the term SDA does not infer that these drugs are selective for serotonin and dopamine receptors, but rather that it is via action at those receptors that they exert their primary effect.

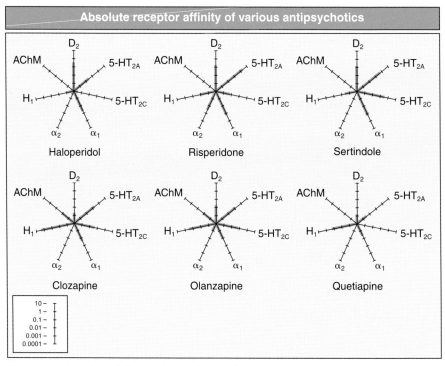

Figure 4.1. Data from [1]. Each line indicates the affinity of that drug for a single receptor. Each of the marks on the lines represent 10 x greater affinity for the receptor. Thus, haloperidol has 1000 x greater affinity for dopamine D_2 receptors than quetiapine.

The use of the novel third generation antipsychotics for maintenance treatment has not yet been fully validated in newly diagnosed or chronic schizophrenic populations by published randomized controlled trials (RCTs) similar to those described in Chapter 3 for the older antipsychotics; however, several long-term treatment comparisons have been carried out.

There are several reasons to make the assumption that third generation antipsychotics may be superior to older antipsychotics in prophylaxis. All antipsychotics investigated so far as part of controlled trials have been shown to be equally effective maintenance treatments. As the third generation are at least as efficacious as first generation antipsychotics in acute treatment, it might follow that they will also be adequate long-term treatments; in addition, all of the newer antipsychotics show a reduced propensity to cause extrapyramidal side effects (EPS) at clinical doses. EPS are one of the major causes of noncompliance. Based on preliminary data it may well be that the third generation antipsychotics will be shown to be better for long-term therapy [2]. Although we still do not know precisely how clozapine exerts its effect, all of the third generation antipsychotics share a high $5\text{-HT}_{2A}/\text{striatal D}_2$ receptor blockade ratio as part of their pharmacodynamic profile. It has been suggested that this is why these drugs exhibit a lower incidence of neurological side effects and secondary negative symptoms at optimal doses [3]. It may be hypothesised that if adverse effects and negative symptoms are indeed minimized with the third generation antipsychotics, then non-compliance and rehospitalization rates will be lower than with first generation antipsychotic maintenance treatment [2].

It is useful to review the pharmacology and early clinical data on each of the newer antipsychotics and then focus on specific areas where the newer antipsychotics may have advantages, for example compliance, side effects, negative symptoms, cognition, and affective symptoms in schizophrenia.

Atypical antipyschotic drugs

Clozapine

Clozapine, the prototypical third generation antipsychotic, has been used since the 1960s for treatment of schizophrenia. However, after reports of several deaths from neutropenia, its use has become restricted. In the UK, it can only be used for patients unresponsive to two other antipsychotics given at an adequate dose for an adequate duration, or those with tardive dyskinesia (TD) or severe extrapyramidal symptoms, and only with blood monitoring. Each patient has to be registered and the drug is only dispensed after a normal white cell count. A count is performed every week for 18 weeks, then every two weeks for the next year, and monthly thereafter. Blood monitoring should also continue for four weeks following withdrawal of treatment. Clozapine is contraindicated in those with previous neutropenia.

Important aspects of the pharmacology of clozapine include its low affinity for the D_2 receptor, with higher affinity at the D_1 and D_4 receptors. Clozapine also binds to the extrastriatal D_2-like receptor, the D_3 receptor. It is thought that the low incidence of EPS is due to the low activity at the D_2 receptor. Clozapine also has antagonistic activity at the 5-HT_{1A}, 5-HT_{2A}, 5-HT_{2C}, and 5-HT_3 receptors. It is postulated that it is the balance between the blockade of these receptors that underlies the clinical efficacy of clozapine in improving positive and negative symptomatology. Clozapine also is an antagonist at

25

the α_1-adrenoceptor and less so at the α_2-adrenoceptor, resulting in sedation and hypotension. Other side effects include hypersalivation, weight gain, tachycardia, sedation, and hypotension. More rarely clozapine can produce seizures (in approximately 1–3% of patients) [4–6] and blood dyscrasias (in about 1–3% of patients). The risk of neutropenia is between 1% and 2%, and in most cases it is reversible; the majority of cases (89%) occur within the first 18 weeks of treatment. Risk of agranulocytosis decreases to 0.07% after the first year of treatment. Agranulocytosis probably results from toxic and immunologic factors. It is this latter potentially fatal side effect that has led to the limits on the use of clozapine and the requirement for blood monitoring in patients receiving clozapine. Interestingly, clozapine does not increase serum prolactin.

Clozapine has been investigated in few RCTs of maintenance therapy, due to the restrictions imposed on its use. In one of the few studies published, Essock *et al* [7] followed up a sample of 227 patients randomized to either clozapine or treatment as usual. They reported that those treated with clozapine had significantly greater reductions in side effects, disruptiveness, hospitalization, and readmission after discharge. Furthermore, the clinical efficacy of clozapine in prevention of relapse has been well established, between one and two years of treatment, and there have been reports of good maintenance efficacy for up to 17 years of treatment [8].

Risperidone

Risperidone was the first of the serotonin–dopamine atypical antipsychotics (SDAs). This drug has high affinity for the 5-HT_{2A} receptor, with a similar affinity at the D_2 receptor to most typical antipsychotics. It is an antagonist at both receptors. In the acute phase of treatment, risperidone appears more effective than haloperidol in terms of improvement in positive and, especially, negative symptom scores. Interestingly, in an analysis of the data from two trials of 513 patients [9], risperidone was also superior to haloperidol at reducing hostility/excitement and anxiety/depression.

The optimal dose of risperidone appears to be between 4 mg and 6 mg per day. At doses higher than 8–12 mg per day risperidone can cause EPSs of tremor, rigidity, and restlessness. Risperidone increases serum prolactin, possibly leading to sexual dysfunction.

Risperidone has been assessed for long-term efficacy and safety in a number of long-term, open-label studies. The earlier data of Mertens *et al* [10], Bressa *et al* [11], and Lindstrom *et al* [12] suggested that long-term therapy with risperidone was associated with a meaningful reduction in psychopathology, amelioration of EPSs, and improved social functioning. The first active comparator controlled study compared risperidone (mean daily dose, 9 mg per day) with haloperidol (mean daily dose, 8.9mg per day) over a 12-month period. There were 91 subjects in the risperidone-treated group and 99 in the haloperidol group. There were similar reductions in symptom ratings in both groups, with a trend in favour of risperidone.

Relapse rates were similar at between 14% and 16% [13]. More recently, a meta-analysis of 11 of the risperidone/conventional antipsychotic comparator RCTs has been performed [14]. That author reported that significantly more patients on risperidone showed clinical improvement than with comparator drugs (57% compared with 52%, respectively) and used significantly less medication for EPSs (22.8% compared with 38.4%, respectively).

Sertindole

As well as high affinity for the 5-HT_{2A} receptor, sertindole is thought to specifically target D_2 receptors in the limbic region, and this has been demonstrated in rats. Sertindole is also a potent alpha1-adrenoceptor antagonist.

Sertindole leads to QTC_2 interval prolongation on electrocardiogram (ECG) This interval represents cardiac ventricular repolarization and prolongation, and has been associated with potentially fatal ventricular tachyarrhythmias, in particular torsades-de-pointes. Therefore, patients need an ECG before starting sertindole and regular ECGs during its use. Caution with concomitant use of local and general anaesthetics is recommended. Early clinical studies have indicated similar EPS rates to those of placebo at clinical doses. Sertindole has been reported not to increase plasma pro-lactin levels with long-term use.

Sertindole has been demonstrated to be effective in the maintenance treatment of schizophrenia. Daniel *et al* [15] performed a 12-month double-blind trial of sertindole 24 mg per day and haloperidol 10 mg per day in 282 stable outpatients with schizo-phrenia. Although the sertindole and haloperidol groups were similar in terms of total positive and negative syndrome scale for schizophrenia (PANSS) scores, there was a trend for enhanced efficacy for sertindole on negative symptoms that did not reach statistical significance. The sertindole group was also less frequently hospital-ized (10 out of 40 compared with 16 out of 142 for haloperidol) and had a lower use of anticholinergic medication (15% compared with 35%, respectively).

Because of safety concerns the manufacturers suspended the use of sertindole pending the accumulation of more safety data. Sertindole is available in the UK on a named-patient basis only, and will not be considered further in this Chapter.

Olanzapine

Olanzapine is a broad-spectrum atypical antipsychotic structurally similar to clozap-ine and demonstrates antagonistic effects at a wide range of doses. Olanzapine has a side-effect profile similar to that of clozapine, but has a higher risk of EPSs than place-bo at doses above 15–20 mg per day. Olanzapine also demonstrates antagonistic effects at a wide range of receptors, but has a higher affinity for D_2 and 5-HT_{2A} recep-tors than clozapine and a lower affinity at the D_1 receptor subtype. In acute phase studies olanzapine is definitely efficacious for positive and secondary negative symptoms, and is superior to haloperidol on overall improvement according to the brief psychiatric rating scale (BPRS) and every other secondary measure [16]. Olanzapine may also be effective for the primary negative symptoms of schizophrenia.

Standard-dose olanzapine (5–15 mg per day) is an effective maintenance treatment for schizophrenia compared with placebo and low-dose olanzapine (1 mg per day) [17]. This was demonstrated in a 46-week extension of acute phase studies. There were 93 patients overall in the standard-dose olanzapine-treated group, 14 patients in the low-dose olanzapine-treated group and 13 patients in the placebo-treated group, respectively. The estimated risk of relapse with olanzapine was 19.6–28.6% for standard dose (5–15 mg per day) compared with 45.5% with low dose (1 mg per day), and the risk of relapse in the placebo-treated group was 69.9%.

Initial data from a meta-analysis of three studies using haloperidol-treated patients as a test group indicates that 80.3% of patients receiving olanzapine maintain their response after one year, compared with 72% of patients treated with haloperidol [18].

Quetiapine

Quetiapine is another broad-spectrum atypical antipsychotic. Quetiapine has a similar receptor binding profile to that of clozapine. Compared with clozapine, quetiapine has a relatively lower affinity for all receptors, with very little affinity for muscarinic receptors. Quetiapine is effective in acute phase studies for the treatment of positive and secondary negative symptoms. In randomized controlled trials, quetiapine has been shown to be more effective than placebo [19,20]. Response rates to quetiapine and chlorpromazine were similar across all symptom domains (mean dose, 407 mg quetiapine compared with 384 mg chlorpromazine). Using the criteria of greater than a 50% reduction in BPRS scores, 65% of quetiapine-treated patients were responders compared with 52% in the chlorpromazine group (p=0.04) [21]. Arvanitis *et al* [19] have reported a dose-ranging study comparing 12 mg of haloperidol with fixed doses of quetiapine between 75 and 750 mg per day, involving a total of 361 patients. At six weeks, the response rates were significantly better than placebo in the haloperidol group and groups treated with a dose of at least 150 mg per day of quetiapine. Response rates between the haloperidol- and quetiapine-treated groups were similar. Further studies have replicated these findings [22] and found that at doses below 250 mg quetiapine is not significantly more effective than placebo [20]. With regard to dosing, it is important to note that in a study of 288 patients with a partial response to fluphenazine, quetiapine at 600 mg per day showed benefits over haloperidol at 20 mg per day. Although in this study mean ratings were similar with a trend in favour of quetiapine, 52% responded to quetiapine versus 38% to haloperidol (p=0.043) [23]. The rates of EPSs with quetiapine are similar to those seen in placebo-treated groups and lower than with the conventional antipsychotic haloperidol group [19–23]. Common side effects with quetiapine include somnolence and dry mouth.

In the open-label extensions of the acute trials 265 responders to quetiapine were considered suitable for one year of treatment. Of these, 33% were still on quetiapine after 12-month follow up, with a sustained level of symptomatic improvement [24]. This is similar to continuation rates in similar trials with olanzapine.

In these long-term studies, quetiapine was well tolerated with up to 75% of respondents to a questionnaire denying any side effects during the previous month [25].

Ziprasidone

Not yet available in the UK, ziprasidone has a high $5\text{-}HT_{2A}$:D_2 receptor blockade ratio and a similarly high affinity for the $5\text{-}HT_{2A}$ receptor to that of other SDAs. It is an agonist at the $5\text{-}HT_{1A}$ receptor. Ziprasidone also has potent affinity for D_3 and moderate affinity for D_4 receptors. It exhibits weak serotonin and noradrenergic reuptake inhibition. Ziprasidone appears to have relatively low levels of side effects. These may include somnolence, headache, and mild weight gain.

An initial clinical trial of ziprasidone versus haloperidol 15 mg per day over four weeks suggested that ziprasidone 160 mg per day was as effective as haloperidol at reducing positive symptom scores but produced fewer extrapyramidal side effects [26]. Further data was reviewed by Tandon *et al* [27]. In two placebo-controlled trials involving 139 and 302 patients over four and six weeks, respectively, the pooled data indicated that treatment with ziprasidone between 80 mg and 160 mg per day was consistently more significantly effective than placebo and lower doses of ziprasidone. Improvements in positive and negative symptoms were similar in magnitude to those seen in patients treated with risperidone, olanzapine or quetiapine. Interestingly, 160 mg ziprasidone was associated with a greater than 30% decrease in depressive symptoms in the subgroup of patients with significant depression at the start of the trials.

Ziprasidone has also been used in a one-year placebo-controlled trial in order to assess its use for relapse prevention. A total of 294 patients were studied and randomized to placebo treatment or ziprasidone between 40 mg and 160 mg per day. Of the patients who were still in the trial at six months (n = 117), only 6% of those on ziprasidone had experienced an exacerbation of their symptoms after one year compared with 35% of the patients treated with placebo (n = 23); this compares favourably with the available data on the older antipsychotics [28; data on file, Pfizer Pharmaceuticals group].

Other agents

Other atypical antipsychotic medications for schizophrenia include amisulpride and zotepine with other newer medications currently in late phase clinical development.

Adverse events

The issue of side effects or adverse events is closely linked to tolerability and acceptability, and therefore to both compliance and relapse prevention. Often the most debilitating and obvious side effects of conventional antipsychotics are motor side effects. As described above, all of the newer antipsychotics demonstrate a lower propensity to cause EPS at clinically effective doses. At these doses, quetiapine and clozapine and, at low doses, olanzapine have rates of EPS similar to placebo treatments [20, 29, 30]. In addition to the classical pseudo-parkinsonian side effects of tremor, bradykinesia, and rigidity, these drugs may provide benefits for patients who suffer from akathisia and tardive dyskinesia.

Akathisia develops in 18–75% of patients treated with typical antipsychotics. Although an early study with clozapine failed to show a significant difference between clozapine and other drugs [31], this was probably due to an inadequate washout time for previous therapy. Later studies have indicated that over a 12-week period there is a striking reduction in akathisia [32, 33], with rates of less than 10%. Indeed, clozapine leads to a reduction in akathisia (from 18–75% to 10%) [33]. Moller *et al* [34] have reported that risperidone at between 4 mg and 8 mg per day produces a significantly lower incidence of akathisia than haloperidol [34]. Olanzapine treatment groups have improved akathisia ratings from baseline [35] and quetiapine shows similar akathisia rates to placebo [20,22].

It is in the area of tardive dyskinesia (TD) that clozapine appears to have the most marked effect. On conventional treatments TD develops in between 5% and 60% of patients, with an increased risk of 3–5% per year of treatment [36–38]. Clozapine treatment has a very low risk of causing TD. Case reports of TD with clozapine treatment are rare [39] and may reflect the natural occupance of TD. Cases of TD have been reported in controlled studies. Gerlach and Peacock [40] reported nine from 100, and Kane *et al* [41] reported two from 28 patients treated for over a year. It is possible, however, that these patients had questionable TD at the outset [42,43]. There is far more evidence supporting a decrease in TD for patients commenced on clozapine. Lieberman *et al* [44] reported a 50% reduction of symptoms over 28 months of treatment in 43% of patients, and Gerlach and Peacock [40] reported a resolution of TD in 54% of patients after five years of clozapine treatment. Furthermore, Tamminga *et al* [45] reported a significant difference in reduction of TD scores in a clozapine group versus a haloperidol-treated group, and that this difference began after about four months of treatment. There have also been case reports of switching to clozapine being effective in reducing tardive dystonia [46].

Given that an increased risk of TD is associated with more profound EPSs at the start of treatment, there are *a priori* reasons for assuming lower rates of TD with all the newer medications. In risperidone-treated groups at less than 10 mg per day there are EPS benefits that increase over time, with a rate of TD at approximately 0.3% per year [12,47]. Additional evidence comes from the large-scale controlled studies with olanzapine, which has a 0.52% one-year risk of TD versus 7.45% for haloperidol (13.5 mg compared with 13.9 mg per day, respectively) [48]. These findings tie in with an early short-term study of quetiapine compared with haloperidol and a longer-term study of ziprasidone compared with placebo. In the quetiapine study, patients treated with higher doses of quetiapine (750 mg per day) showed a greater improvement in abnormal involuntary movements compared with the haloperidol-treated group. Long-term data with quetiapine has found a one-year risk of TD of 0.7–1% [49]. In the zisprasidone study, placebo levels of tardive dyskinesia were noted up to one year of treatment [28, data on file, Pfizer Pharmaceuticals Group].

As concern over EPS has waned, the weight gain associated with antipsychotic use has gained increasing importance. Weight gain has long been associated with the use of typical antipsychotics particularly phenothiazines [50]. A recent meta-analysis of extant clinical trials has compared the weight gain caused by the newer antipsychotics with the older antipsychotics [51]. In this study weight gain was estimated at 10 weeks of treatment with the relevant antipsychotic medication. For risperidone the mean weight gain at 10 weeks was estimated to be 2kg, (Confidence Interval [CI] 1.61 to 2.39), for clozapine 3.99kg (CI 2.72 to 5.26), for olanzapine, 3.51kg, (CI 3.29 to 3.73) and for ziprasidone 0.04kg (CI -0.49 to 0.57). This compares with 2.1kg (CI 0.85 to 3.35) for chlorpromazine and 0.48kg (CI 0.07 to 1.03) for haloperidol. Although not included in this analysis, at 9-13 weeks of treatment, quetiapine was associated with a mean weight gain of 1.58 kg [52], however a recent longitudinal study of quetiapine-treated patients has indicated that there is a mean net weight loss of 1.53 kg after treatment with quetiapine for 52 weeks. After 104 weeks of treatment a weight gain of 1.94 kg was noted. Thus in this group treated with quetiapine there was no net weight gain over two years of treatment. [53].

The rates of other side effects may vary between each of the newer drugs, although fully adequate comparison studies remain to be published. A comparison based on the available literature is shown in Table 4.2 [54].

Side effect profiles of antipsychotic agents						
Side effects	Typicals	Clozapine	Risperidone	Olanzapine	Quetiapine	Ziprasidone
Anticholinergic	± to +++	+++	±	+	±	±
Orthostatic hypotension	± to +++	+++	+	±	+	±
Prolactin elevation	++ to +++	o	++	±	±	±
QT prolongation	± to +	+	± to +	± to +	± to +	± to +
Sedation	+ to +++	+++	+	++	++	+
Seizures	±	++ to +++	±	±	±	±
Weight gain	± to ++	+++	+ to ++	+++	± to +	±
o, absent; ±, minimal; +, mild; ++, moderate; +++, severe.						

Table 4.2. Adapted with permission from [54].

Compliance

Compliance with treatment is undoubtably crucial in psychiatric illnesses and is one of the most frequent reasons for readmission to hospital. Noncompliance may be related to a number of factors, including the nature of illness, the degree of insight, and the frequency and acceptability of side effects [55]. Rates of noncompliance are high even in clinical trial populations as many as 30% become noncompliant within one year [56]. A quarter to two-thirds of patients who discontinue medication treatment cite medication side effects as the major reason for their noncompliance. Noncompliance rates may be reduced by vigorous strategies to reduce side effects, for example switching patients onto the newer antipsychotics [57].

Patients on clozapine have low non-compliance rates (approximately 7%) [54], supporting the findings above and the notion that compliance may be enhanced in patients receiving the newer antipsychotics. It has been hypothesised that the reasons for this reduced rate may be a combination of the fewer EPS seen with clozapine and the frequent contact required for blood monitoring [58]. The commitment to blood monitoring has been suggested by some authors [59] to lead to a 30–50% dropout rate from clozapine therapy, however, and thus the effect may be primarily mediated by the low EPS profile of clozapine. All of the newer antipsychotics share with clozapine a lower liklihood of causing EPS. Therefore, it is possible that compliance with the newer drugs will be higher. Data on dropout rates from the typical antipsychotic controlled clinical trials of the newer antipsychotics support this assumption. In a meta-analysis of risperidone RCTs [14], risperidone-treated groups were significantly less likely to drop out than groups treated with conventional antipsychotics (29.1% compared with 33.9%, respectively). In one trial comparing risperidone with haloperidol, 52% of risperidone-treated patients dropped out of treatment versus 63% for haloperidol, and risperidone-treated patients stayed on treatment for longer before dropping out [12]. Tollefson *et al* [16] reported that in the acute phase of treatment 53% of patients treated with haloperidol (mean daily dose, 11.8 mg) and only 33% of patients treated with olanzapine (mean daily dose, 13.2 mg) dropped out of treatment. In a comparison of chlorpromazine and quetiapine, patients receiving quetiapine were less than half as likely to drop out of treatment because of an adverse event [19]. In comparison with haloperidol, patients treated with quetiapine were four times less likely to drop out of treatment because of adverse events [20]. Although total dropout rates did not differ in these two studies, a treatment satisfaction survey of patients maintained on quetiapine reported a very high rate of satisfaction with and acceptability of quetiapine, with 97% of the study group preferring quetiapine over their previous medication treatment [25].

Negative symptoms

It is postulated that clozapine has an almost unique action against the negative symptoms of schizophrenia, out of proportion to its effect on positive symptoms [60,61], but the evidence for this is by no means clear. Tandon *et al* [62] found that the improvement in negative symptoms covaried with the improvement in positive symptoms, and Hagger *et al* [63] found no improvement in negative symptoms. A more recent finding is that clozapine, in a comparison with haloperidol, has a significant effect on negative symptoms in patients with nondeficit schizophrenia, but not in those with deficit schizophrenia (ie, those with enduring negative symptoms) [64,65]. It has therefore been suggested that the apparent beneficial effect of clozapine on negative symptoms may simply be a reflection of its reduced tendency to cause EPS [66]. The weight of current evidence suggests that clozapine has an excellent effect on these secondary but not primary negative symptoms [67]. All of the newer antipsychotics appear to have an effect on secondary negative symptoms. Available trials have indicated a modest but significant advantage for newer medications over conventional antipsychotics in negative symptom improvement [13,15,16]. The data from trials of risperidone, olanzapine and quetiapine have been assessed using a path-analytical approach that attempts to control for changes in negative symptoms score which are simply related to a reduction in adverse effects. At 6 mg per day risperidone has a direct effect on PANSS negative symptoms in chronic schizophrenia [34]. Olanzapine has been reported to have an effect on core primary negative symptoms at doses of 15 mg±2.5 mg per day [68]. In a path analysis of data from 1106 patients with schizophrenia in three acute placebo controlled trials, quetiapine produced a greater improvement in negative symptoms (assessed by SANS total score) than placebo. Of this superior efficacy over placebo, 44.2% was attributable to a direct effect of quetiapine on negative symptoms (personal communication, AstraZeneca). Path-analytical methods have limitations, however, and further work will need to performed in this area with careful delineation of primary and secondary negative symptoms.

Cognition

The older antipsychotics have limited impact on the neurocognitive deficits, which are a core feature of schizophrenia, are apparent at the onset of illness, and may deteriorate during the first few years of illness, although inconsistent long-term improvements have been noted [69,70]. There has been increasing interest in the role that newer antipsychotics may have in ameliorating these problems, which are linked to poor outcome and future unemployment. Clozapine may lead to improvements in attention, memory, and executive function over 6–12 months [71]. Risperidone appears to improve frontal function and spatial working memory versus haloperidol [72]. Olanzapine improves a variety of measures of function including psychomotor speed, verbal fluency, and memory [73]. It has been reported that quetiapine improves attentional performance to the level of that seen in a matched control group over two months of treatment [74]. A preliminary study comparing quetiapine (n = 26) and haloperidol (n = 15) in a randomized, double-blind trial demonstrated that patients treated with quetiapine showed significant improvements in overall cognitive performance, verbal fluency and verbal contextual memory [75].

It is still not clear how relevant the modest improvements reported in these studies are to long-term outcome. However, it is likely that the benefits will become increasingly apparent as longer term studies are performed.

Affective symptoms and use in other disorders

Patients with schizophrenia are significantly more likely than the general population to suffer from other psychiatric disorders, for example depression, and conventional antipsychotics are used to treat other psychotic disorders outside of schizophrenia. It is useful, therefore, to look at the possible benefits of the newer medications in limiting comorbid disorders and the possibility of using them outside of schizophrenia.

Clozapine has efficacy in a number of other disorders where traditionally typical antipsychotics have been used. Clozapine has been reported to be effective in patients with treatment-resistant schizoaffective or manic illnesses [76]. In one study [77] clozapine reduced baseline mania ratings by greater than 50% in 72% of a group of patients suffering from either mania or schizoaffective disorder, and 32% had a significant improvement in BPRS scores. The latter finding was more frequent in the bipolar and the nonrapid cycling patients [77]. In depressive disorders clozapine has a more equivocal response. Although seemingly effective against depressive symptoms occurring comorbidly with schizophrenia [78], there has been little work showing a particular use for clozapine in treatment-refractory depression [79,80].

Conventional antipsychotics may both improve and contribute towards depressive symptoms. Clozapine reduces both depressive features and suicidality [78]. Risperidone produces significantly greater reduction in anxiety/depression subscales compared with haloperidol [9], as does quetiapine (personal communication, AstraZeneca). Olanzapine has significant antidepressant effects in schizophrenia compared with haloperidol [81].

The finding that clozapine, in patients resistant to previous classical antipsychotic treatment, reduces the incidence of suicidality (suicidal ideation, planning, attempts, and suicide completion) from that seen at baseline is of particular interest in the UK because of recent government targets. Meltzer and Okayli [78] reported a reduction of suicidality in 40% of their patients and the number of patients with no reported suicidality increased from 54–88%. Further evidence for decreased suicidality is that the rates of suicide among the 50,000 plus patients in the USA who have received clozapine is one-tenth of that seen in the general schizophrenic population (0.09% compared with 0.8%, respectively) [78,82]. There is an ongoing randomised trial comparing the effects of clozapine and olanzapine on suicidality and suicide in schizophrenia. The data from this study (InterSePT) should be ready in 2001/2002 [83]. In the quetiapine clinical trials programme the incidence of suicidality was 0.3% in patients treated with quetiapine compared with 0.5% for risperidone and 1.3% for haloperidol [84].

Pharmacoeconomics

The high cost of clozapine and other atypical antipsychotics, when compared with classical antipsychotics, has sparked an increasing interest in analysing the cost of drug treatment as a function of the cost of total care (ie, number of hospitalizations, residential care, number of outpatient attendances, and intensity of community input). The area of clozapine pharmacoeconomics has been extensively reviewed by Fitton and Benfield [85]. In summary, in 1987 schizophrenia was estimated to directly and indirectly cost the UK, £1,600 million of which the annual direct cost is estimated to be £1,669 per patient. In the USA it is estimated that the annual direct cost of treatment-resistant schizophrenia is US$11,300 million to US$22,600 million.

Analyses of cost effectiveness of clozapine treatment in the USA indicated that, on the whole, clozapine was more expensive during the initiation of treatment, but that over and after the first year there were substantial savings that were more marked in insured or self-funding patients than in those paid for with public funds. These savings were mainly due to a reduced number of days in hospital for the clozapine-treated groups [86]. A similar analysis in the UK indicated that clozapine treatment was either slightly cheaper or cost the same as conventional treatment, with an estimated saving to the National Health Service of £91 per patient per year [87].

The largest part of the savings with clozapine appears to be in reducing the amount of time that patients with schizophrenia spend in hospital. It is therefore interesting to note that during one year of treatment with risperidone the number of days that the patients spent in an inpatient bed (bed-days) reduced to 13 from 54 bed-days on the treatment the patients had been receiving in the year before starting risperidone [88]. Olanzapine has been reported to lead to cost savings in the US, of $9,400 per patient per year in comparison to haloperidol [89]. For quetiapine recent UK data has suggested a reduction in bed-days from 45 days to 30 days, and a cost saving of £1,600 per patient per year [90]. A study comparing the costs of risperidone versus haloperidol treatment in Australia [91] has indicated that risperidone cost two-thirds as much as haloperidol per expected favourable outcome and five-sixths the total cost of haloperidol over two years.

Conclusion

Although the evidence that the newer antipsychotics are more effective in the maintenance treatment and prevention of relapse in schizophrenia is preliminary, it is becoming increasingly clear that the rational use of these medications offer mild-to-moderate advantages over older antipsychotic medication in a number of different spheres of schizophrenia treatment. Cumulatively, the benefits may be substantial. The data presented here indicates that the newer antipsychotics offer enhanced efficacy for positive and negative symptoms and reduced short- and long-term side effects, are more acceptable to patients suffering from schizophrenia, and offer improvements in mood and cognition in comparison with older antipsychotics. These effects may be additive or synergistic, combining to allow patients to enter more into the mainstream of rehabilitation, psychological therapies, and employment. This could lead to a 'snowball' effect of greatly enhanced improvement in quality of life for people suffering from a lifelong and debilitating illness.

References

1. Schotte A, Janssen PF, Gommeren W *et al*. **Risperidone compared with new and reference antipsychotic drugs: in vitro and in vivo receptor binding.** *Psychopharmacol* (Berlin) 1996; **124**(1-2):57–73.

2. Weiden P, Aquila R, Standard J. **Atypical antipsychotic drugs and long-term outcome in schizophrenia.** *J Clin Psychiatry* 1996; **57**(suppl. 11):53–60.

3. Kapur S, Remington G. **Serotonin–dopamine interaction and its relevance to schizophrenia.** *Am J Psychiatry* 1996; **153**:466–476.

4. Erlandsen C. **Clozapine for schizophrenia. Clinical effect, financial considerations and quality requirements.** *Nord J Psychiatry* 2000; **54**(2):143-148.

5. Devinsky O, Honigfeld G, Patin J. **Clozapine-related seizures.** *Neurology* 1991;**41**(3):369-71.

6 Pacia SV, Devinsky O. **Clozapine-related seizures: experience with 5629 patients.** *Neurology* 1994;**44**(12):2247-9.

7. Essock SM, Hargreaves WA, Covell NH *et al*. **Clozapine's effectiveness for patients in state hospitals: results from a randomized trial.** *Psychopharmacol Bull* 1996; **32**(4):683–697.

8. Travis MJ. **Clozapine: A review.** *J Serotonin Res* 1997; **4**(2):125–144.

9. Marder SR, Davis JM, Chouinard G. **The effects of risperidone on the five dimensions of schizophrenia derived by factor analysis: combined results of the North American trials.** *J Clin Psychiatry* 1997; **58**(12):538–546.

10. Mertens C. **Long term treatment of schizophrenic patients with risperidone.** *Biol Psychiatry* 1991; **29**:413S–414S.

11. Bressa GM, Bersani G, Meco G *et al*. **One years follow-up study with risperidone in chronic schizophrenia.** *New Trends Exp Clin Psychiatry* 1991; **7**(4):169–177.

12. Lindstrom E, Eriksson B, Hellgren A *et al*. **Efficacy and safety of risperidone in the long-term treatment of patients with schizophrenia.** *Clin Ther* 1995; **17**(3):402–412.

13. Lopez-Ibor JJ, Ayuso JL, Gutiérrez M *et al*. **Risperidone in the treatment of chronic schizophrenia:multicenter study comparative to haloperidol [Spanish].** *Actas Luso Esp Neurol Psiquiatr Cienc Afines* 1996; **24**(4):165–172.

14. Song F. **Risperidone in the treatment of schizophrenia: a meta-analysis of randomized controlled trials.** *J Psychopharmacol* 1997; **11**(1):65–71.

15. Daniel DG, Wozniak P, Mack RJ *et al*. **Long-term efficacy and safety comparison of sertindole and haloperidol in the treatment of schizophrenia. The Sertindole Study Group.** *Psychopharmacol Bull* 1998; **34**(1):61–69.

16. Tollefson GD, Beasley CM Jr, Tran PV *et al*. **Olanzapine versus haloperidol in the treatment of schizophrenia and schizoaffective and schizophreniform disorders: results of an international collaborative trial.** *Am J Psychiatry* 1997; **154**(4):457–465.

17. Dellva MA, Tran P, Tollefson GD *et al*. **Standard olanzapine versus placebo and ineffective-dose olanzapine in the maintenance treatment of schizophrenia [see comments].** *Psychiatr Serv* 1997; **48**(12):1571–1577.

18. Tran PV, Dellva MA, Tollefson GD *et al*. **Oral olanzapine versus oral haloperidol in the maintenance treatment of schizophrenia and related psychoses.** *Br J Psychiatry* 1998; **172**:499–505.

19. Arvanitis LA, Miller BG, and the Seroquel Trial 13 Study Group. **Multiple fixed doses of 'Seroquel' (quetiapine) in patients with acute exacerbation of schizophrenia: a comparison with haloperidol and placebo.** *Biol Psychiatry* 1997; **42**(4):233–246.

20. Small JG, Hirsch SR, Arvanitis LA *et al*. **Quetiapine in Patients with Schizophrenia.** *Arch Gen Psychiatr* 1997; **54**:549–557.

21. Peuskens J, Link CG. **A comparison of quetiapine and chlorpromazine in the treatment of schizophrenia.** *Acta Psychiatr Scand* 1997; **96**(4):265–273.

22. Copolov DL, Link CGG, Kowalcyk B. **A multicentre, double-blind, randomised comparison of quetiapine (ICI 204,636, 'Seroquel') and haloperidol in schizophrenia.** *Psychol Med* 2000; **30**:95–106.

23. Emsley RA, Raniwalla J, Bailey PJ *et al*. **A comparison of the effects of quetiapine ('Seroquel') and haloperidol in schizophrenic patients with a history of and a demonstrated, partial response to conventional antipsychotic treatment.** *Int Clin Psychopharmacol* 2000; **15**:121–131.

24. Rak I, Raniwalla J. **Maintenance of Long-term efficacy with seroquel (quetiapine).** *Schizophr Res* 2000; **41**:205.

25. Hellewell JSE, Kalali AH, Langham SJ *et al*. **Patient satisfaction and acceptability of long-term treatment with quetiapine.** *Int J Psychiatr Clin Pract* 1999; **3**:105–113.

26. Goff DC, Posever T, Herz L *et al*. **An exploratory haloperidol-controlled dose-finding study of ziprasidone in hospitalized patients with schizophrenia or schizoaffective disorder.** *J Clin Psychopharmacol* 1998; **18**(4):296–304.

27. Tandon R, Harrigan E, Zorn SH *et al*. **Ziprasidone: A novel antipsychotic with unique pharmacology and therapeutic potential.** *J Serotonin Res* 1997; **4**:159–177.

28. Arato M, O'Connor R, Meltzer H *et al*. *The Ziprasidone extended use in Schizophrenia (ZEUS) Study: A prospective, double blind, placebo controlled, 1 year clinical trial.* Data on file: Pfizer Pharmaceutical Group; 1999.

29. Goldstein JM. **Atypical antipsychotic drugs: beyond acute psychosis, new directions.** *Emerg Drugs* 1999; **4**:127–151

30. *Physicians Desk Reference 55th Edition*, 2001; Medical Economics Company; pp1788–1793

31. Cohen BM, Keck PE, Satlin A *et al*. **Prevalence and severity of akathisia in patients on clozapine.** *Biol Psychiatry* 1991; **15**(29):1215–1219.

32. Safferman AZ, Lieberman JA, Pollack S *et al*. **Clozapine and Akathisia.** *Biol Psychiatry* 1992; **31**:753–754.

33. Chengappa KN, Shelton MD, Baker RW *et al*. **The prevalence of akathisia in patients receiving stable doses of clozapine.** *J Clin Psychiatry* 1994; **55**(4):142–145.

34. Moller HJ, Bauml J, Ferrero F *et al*. **Risperidone in the treatment of schizophrenia: results of a study of patients from Germany, Austria and Switzerland.** *Eur Arch Psychiatry Clin Neurosci* 1996; **247**:291–296.

37

35. Beasley CM, Tollefson GD, Tran PV. **Safety of olanzapine.** *J Clin Psychiatry* 1996; **10**:13–17.

36. Malhotra AK, Litman RE, Pickar D *et al.* **Adverse effects of antipsychotics drugs.** *Drug Saf* 1993; **9**:429–436.

37. Fleischhacker WW, Whitworth AB. **Adverse effects of antipsychotic drugs.** *Curr Opin Psychiatry* 1994; **7**:71–75.

38. Jeste DV, Caliguri MP, Paulsen JS *et al.* **Risk of tardive dyskinesia in older patients: a prospective longitudinal study of 266 outpatients.** *Arch Gen Psychiatry* 1995; **52**(9):756–765.

39. de Leon J, Moral L, Camunas C. **Clozapine and jaw dyskinesia: a case report.** *J Clin Psychiatry* 1991; **52**:494–495.

40. Gerlach J, Peacock L. **Motor and mental side effects of clozapine.** *J Clin Psychiatry* 1994; **55**(suppl. B):107–109.

41. Kane JM, Safferman AZ, Pollack S *et al.* **Clozapine, negative symptoms and extrapyramidal side effects.** *J Clin Psychiatry* 1994; **55**(suppl. B):74–77.

42. Wagstaff AJ, Bryson HM. **Clozapine: A review of its Pharmacological properties and therapeutic use in patients with schizophrenia who are unresponsive to or intolerent of classical antipsychotic agents.** *CNS Drugs* 1995; **4**(5):370–400.

43. Cunningham-Owens DG. **Adverse effects of antipsychotic agents. Do newer agents offer advantages?** *Drugs* 1996; **51**(6):895–930.

44. Lieberman JA, Saltz BL, Johns GA *et al.* **The effects of clozapine on tardive dyskinesia.** *Br J Psychiatry* 1991; **158**:503–510.

45. Tamminga CA, Thaker GK, Moran M *et al.* **Clozapine in tardive dyskinesia: observations for human and animal model studies.** *J Clin Psychiatry* 1994; **55**(suppl. B):102–106.

46. Shapleske J, Mickay AP, McKenna PJ *et al.* **Successful treatment of tardive dystonia with clozapine and clonazepam.** *Br J Psychiatry* 1996; **168**(4):516–518.

47. Gutierrez-Esteinou R, Grebb JA. **Resperidone: an analysis of the first three years in general use.** *Int Clin Psychopharmacol* 1997; **12**(suppl. 4):S3–S10.

48. Beasley CM Jr, Dellva MA, Tamura RN *et al.* **Randomised double-blind comparison of the incidence of tardive dyskinesia in patients with schizophrenia during long-term treatment with olanzapine or haloperidol.** *Br J Psychiatry* 1999; **174**:23–30.

49. Glazer WM, Morgenstern H, Pultz JA *et al.* Poster presented at the 10th Biennial Winter Workshop on Schizophrenia. Davos, Switzerland, 5–11 Feb 2000.

50. Bernstein JG. **Induction of obesity by psychotropic drugs.** *Annals of the New York Academy of Science* 1987; **499**:203-215.

51. Allison DB, Mentore JL, Heo M *et al.* **Antipsychotic-induced weight gain: a comprehensive research synthesis.** *Am J Psych* 1999; **156**(11):1686-96).

52. Rak IW, Jones AM, Raniwalla J *et al.* **Weight Changes in patients treated with seroquel (quetiapine).** *Schizophr Res* 2000; **41**:206. Poster presentation (*see* ref. 49).

53. Hellewell JSE, Westhead EK. **Safety During Long-Term Exposure to Quetiapine.** Presented at the American College of Neuropsychopharmacology Annual Meeting in Puerto Rico, 10–14 Dec 2000.

54. Jibson MD, Tandon R. **New atypical antipsychotic medications.** *J Psychiatr Res* 1998; **32**(3/4):215–228.

55. Lindstrom LH. **Long term clinical and social outcome studies in schizophrenia in relation to the cognitive and emotional side effects of antipsychotic drugs.** *Acta Psychiatr Scand* 1994; 380(suppl.):74–76.

56. Kane JM. **Compliance issues in outpatient treatment.** *J Clin Psychopharmacol* 1985; 5:22S–27S.

57. Fenton WS, Blyler CR, Heinssen RK. **Determinants of Medication Compliance in Schizophrenia: Empirical and Clinical Findings.** *Schizophr Bull* 1997; 23(4):637–651.

58. Carpenter WT Jr. **Maintenance Therapy of Persons with schizophrenia.** *J Clin Psychiatry* 1996; 57(suppl. 9):10–18.

59. Hirsch SR, Puri BK. **Clozapine: progress in treating refractory schizophrenia.** *Br Med J* 1993; 306:1427–1428.

60. Meltzer HY. **Pharmacologic treatment of negative symptoms.** In: *Negative Schizophrenic symptoms: Pathophysiology and Clinical Implications.* Edited by JF Greden and R Tandon. Washington: American Psychiatric Press; 1990.

61. Meltzer HY. **The effect of clozapine and other atypical drugs on negative symptoms.** In: *Negative Versus Positive Schizophrenia.* Edited by A Marneros, NC Andreasen and MT Tsuang. Berlin: Springer-Verlag.

62. Tandon R, Ribeiro SC, De Quardo JR *et al.* **Covariance of positive and negative symptoms during neuroleptic treatment in schizophrenia: a replication.** *Biol Psychiatry* 1993; 34(7):495–497.

63. Hagger C, Buckley P, Kenny ST *et al.* **Improvement in cognitive functions and psychiatric symptoms in treatment refractory schizophrenic patients receiving clozapine.** *Biol Psychiatry* 1993; 34:702–712.

64. Breier A, Buchanan RW, Waltrip RW *et al.* **The effects of clozapine on plasma norepinephrine: relationship to clinical efficacy.** *Neuropsychopharmacol* 1994; 10:1–7.

65. Conley R, Gounaris C, Tamminga C. **Clozapine response varies in deficit versus non-deficit schizophrenic subjects.** *Biol Psychiatry* 1994; 35:746–747.

66. Kane JM, Safferman AZ, Pollack S *et al.* **Clozapine, negative symptoms, and extrapyramidal side effects.** *J Clin Psychiatry* 1994; 55(suppl. B):74–77.

67. Carpenter WTJ, Conley RR, Buchanan RW *et al.* **Patient response and resource management: another view of clozapine treatment of schizophrenia.** *Am J Psychiatry* 1995; 152:827–832.

68. Tollefson GD, Sanger TM. **Negative symptoms: a path analytic approach to a double-blind, placebo- and haloperidol-controlled clinical trial with olanzapine.** *Am J Psychiatry* 1997; 154(4):466–474.

69. Meltzer HY, Thompson PA, Lee MA *et al.* **Neuropsychologic deficits in schizophrenia: relation to social function and effect of antipsychotic treatment.** *Neuropsychopharmacology* 1996; 14(suppl. 3):27S–33S.

70. Bilder RM. **Neurocognitive impairment in schizophrenia and how it affects treatment options.** *Can J Psychiatry* 1997; 42(3):255–264.

71. Lee MA, Thompson PA, Meltzer HY. **Effects of clozapine on cognitive function in schizophrenia.** *J Clin Psychiatry* 1994; 55(suppl. B):82–87.

72. Gallhofer B, Bauer U, Lis S *et al.* **Cognitive dysfunction in schizophrenia:comparison of treatment with atypical antipsychotic agents and conventional neuroleptic drugs.** *Eur Neuropsychopharmacol* 1996; 6(suppl. 2):S13–S20.

73. McGurk SR, Meltzer HY. **The effects of atypical antipsychotic drugs on cognitive functioning in schizophrenia.** *Schizophr Res* 1998; 29:160.

74. Sax KW, Strakowski SM, Keck PE Jr. **Attentional improvement following quetiapine fumarate treatment in schizophrenia.** *Schizophr Res* 1998; **33**(3):151–155.
75. Velligan DI, Newcomer J, Pultz J *et al.* **Changes in cognitive functioning with quetiapine fumerate versus haloperidol.** American Psychiatric Association Meeting, Washington, USA, 15–20 May 1999; Abstract and poster.
76. Kimmel SE, Calabrese JR, Woyshville MJ *et al.* **Clozapine in treatment-refractory mood disorders.** *J Clin Psychiatry* 1994; **55**(suppl. B):91–93.
77. Calabrese JR, Kimmel SE, Woyshville MJ *et al.* **Clozapine for treatment-refractory mania.** *Am J Psychiatry* 1996; **156**(6):759–764.
78. Meltzer HY, G Okayli. **Reduction of suicidlity during clozapine treatment of neuroleptic-resistant schizophrenia: impact on risk benefit assessment.** *Am J Psychiatry* 1995; **152**:183–190.
79. Banov MD, Zarate CAJ, Tohen M *et al.* **Clozapine therapy in refractory affective disorders: polarity predicts response in long-term follow up.** *J Clin Psychiatry* 1994; **55**(7):295–300.
80. Rothschild AJ. **Management of psychotic, treatment resistant depression.** *Psychiatr Clin North Am* 1996; **19**(2):237–252.
81. Tollefson GD, Sanger TM, Lu Y *et al.* **Depressive signs and symptoms in schizophrenia: a prospective blinded trial of olanzapine and haloperidol [published erratum appears in Arch Gen Psychiatry 1998; 55:1052].** *Arch Gen Psychiatry* 1998; **55**(3):250–258.
82. Cohen LJ, Test MA, Brown RL. **Suicide and schizophrenia: data from a prospective community treatment study [published erratum appears in Am J Psychiatry 1990; 147:1110].** *Am J Psychiatry* 1990; **147**(5):602–607.
83. Meltzer HY. **Suicide and schizophrenia: clozapine and the InterSept study. International Clozaril/Leponex Suicide Prevention Trial.** *J Clin Psychiatry* 1999; **60**(suppl 12):47–50.
84. Meltzer HY, Dev VJ. **Suicidality during quetiapine treatment.** Poster presented at the 22nd Collegium Internationale Neuropsychopharmacologicum Congress, Brussels, Belgium, 9–13 July 2000.
85. Fitton A, Benfield P. **Clozapine: An appraisal of its Pharmacoeconomic Benefits in the Treatment of Schizophrenia.** *Pharmacoeconomics* 1993; **4**(2):131–156.
86. Reid WH, Mason M, Toprac M. **Savings in hospital bed-days related to treatment with clozapine.** *Hosp Community Psychiatry* 1994; **45**(3):261–264.
87. Davies LM, Drummond MF. **Assessment of costs and benefits for treatment resistant schizophrenia in the UK.** *Br J Psychiatry* 1993; **162**:38–42.
88. Addington DE, Jones B, Bloom D *et al.* **Reduction of hospital days in chronic schizophrenic patients treated with risperidone: a retrospective study.** *Clin Ther* 1993; **15**(5):917–926.
89. Tunis SL, Crogham T, Heilman DK, *et al.* **Reliability, validity and application of the Medical Outcomes Study 36 – Item Short Form Health Survey (SF – 36) in schizophrenic patients treated with olanzapine versus haloperidol.** *Medical Care* 1999; **37**(7) 678–691.
90. Lynch J, Morrison J, Graves N, *et al.* **The health economic implications of treatments with quetiapine: an audit of long-term treatment for patients with chronic schizophrenia.** *Eur Psy* 2001; **16**;307–312.
91. Davies A, Adena MA, Keks NA *et al.* **Risperidone versus haloperidol: I. Meta-analysis of efficacy and safety.** *Clin Ther* 1998; **20**(1):58–71.

Chapter 5

The role of psychosocial interventions in preventing relapse

Introduction

Increasingly, the importance of psychosocial interventions in preventing relapse is becoming recognised with evidence that relapse rates can be reduced by as much as 50% by psychosocial treatment [1]. Such interventions include family therapy, social, cognitive and occupational rehabilitation, cognitive-behaviour therapy (CBT), medication compliance, and models of early intervention. They are not proposed as alternatives to medication, but should be used as adjunctive therapies. The integration of pharmacological and psychosocial treatments in our provision of services echoes the growing recognition that social and psychological factors interact strongly with biological factors in predicting the course and outcome of schizophrenia [2]. Individuals diagnosed with schizophrenia have complex and multidimensional difficulties which need to be addressed: relationships with their environmental and social networks; understanding of, and attitudes towards, their illness and symptoms; management of disabilities in the cognitive, occupational and social spheres; and the secondary emotional disturbances often experienced, for example substance abuse, depression, and anxiety. Recently, special emphasis has been given to implementing 'early intervention' services in an effort to prevent the deteriorating course of the disorder and preventing relapse. In addition, primary carers often experience substantial burden of care that in turn has implications for the patient's own mental health. All of these factors can affect relapse rates independently of medication, and are the focus of the interventions described below.

Family interventions

The impact of caring for a severely mentally ill relative can be quite substantial [3]. While families do not 'cause' schizophrenia, the burden of care affects the quality of the resulting relationship between carer and patient, that in turn impacts on the course of the illness after onset. The concept of expressed emotion (EE) was initially formulated as an index of the emotional climate within the home environment [4], and is now used to assess the quality of the relationship between patient and relative. An indisputable relationship between EE and relapse has been established, with the critical toxic dimensions pertaining to the frequency of critical comments about the patient, the presence of hostility, and the magnitude of emotional over involvement. In contrast, warmth and positive remarks may have a protective factor. Nine-month

41

relapse rates for patients returning to high EE families across 25 studies was found to be 50%, compared with 21% for low EE environments [5].

Therefore, an important focus in family interventions is to reduce levels of EE, although other therapeutic ingredients are also added (*see* Table 5.1). Overall, there is powerful evidence that family interventions improve outcome, as measured by relapse rates [6]: typically, nine-month relapse rates decrease to less than 20%, compared with 50% in high EE families receiving standard care. Many research groups, in several different cultures, have replicated this. Tarrier and Barrowclough [7] found that even eight years after intervention positive effects were still apparent. Nevertheless, there is evidence that a sizeable number of families either refuse intervention or drop out at an early stage. No strong evidence has emerged for the efficacy of one type of therapy over another, although psychodynamic and purely educational approaches, short-term treatments (of less than three months duration), and interventions that include neither the patient nor the clinical team seem to be unhelpful.

Not all patients live at home, and the relationships between patients and staff carers are subject to the same sorts of factors, despite their seemingly different roles to relatives. For example, Herzog [8] found that 65% of staff on a psychiatric ward had high EE attitudes to one or more patients. There is now some tentative evidence that individuals in care settings with high EE also have poor a outcome [9]. This work suggests that mental health teams need to consider investing in training, supervision and support of their staff carers to reduce the potentially negative effects of the high demands being made of them, in terms of both staff burnout and poor patient outcome.

Beneficial therapeutic elements of family interventions	
Components	**Aims**
Psychoeducation	Increasing understanding of schizophrenia, role of medication and issues of side effects. This should be done over several sessions and include both verbal and written material
Problem solving	Focusing on immediate day to day problems faced by families; stress management
Communication and skills training	Improving communication skills, reducing friction and helping negotiation; teaching coping skills
Emotional processing	Helping awareness of emotional issues and giving emotional support
Cognitive reappraisal	Changing maladaptive attributions of the patient's problems, normalizing extreme emotions and potentially lowering expectations

Table 5.1.

Although family interventions are undoubtedly helpful, over two-thirds of patients will eventually relapse. There are therefore still short-term interventions in the context of problems that for many relatives and patients will last a lifetime. Long-term support by mental health teams is necessary throughout the lifecycle, with some degree of continuity of care. In addition, respite from care is a well-documented requirement but it has been more commonly provided for those caring for the elderly than for the severely mentally ill. Lastly, despite the demonstrated cost savings of family interventions (eg, a saving of 26.2% on mean costs per patient in the Tarrier *et al* study [10]), they have so far failed to be integrated into routine practice and remain an effective but underused treatment.

Rehabilitation

The focus of rehabilitative therapies tends to be on the social, cognitive and occupational disabilities exhibited by individuals with schizophrenia. Historically, such therapies have tended to fall into the following three categories: social skills training, cognitive remediation, and occupational therapy.

Social skills training

Social skills training (SST) aims to remediate the interpersonal deficits demonstrated by individuals with schizophrenia that militate against the ability to integrate into society and therefore contribute to poor long-term outcome. The evidence regarding the efficacy of SST is mixed and wide variations in both the form and the length of interventions make it difficult to draw firm conclusions. SST that involves structured educational methods combining social reinforcement, modelling and role-play appears to be relatively successful [11] and maintained for long periods [12]. One study showed that SST increased social adjustment, in addition to reducing symptoms and relapse rates [13].

However, a meta-analytic review of 23 studies concluded that, although SST is associated with improved interpersonal functioning and lower social anxiety in specific role-play tests, generalization of skills and community functioning over a longer timespan is less robust [14].

Cognitive remediation

Many patients diagnosed with schizophrenia complain of cognitive deficits, for example the inability to concentrate, which may be so severe that it affects every aspect of day-to-day life. There is some evidence that these deficits may have more influence than symptoms on current and future social functioning [15], in discharge destination [16], and treatment [17] and vocational-treatment outcomes [18]; therefore, reducing cognitive deficits has the potential to significantly increase the patient's quality of life and reduce dependence on psychiatric care. Cognitive remediation attempts to reduce deficits by improving patients' performance on a variety of cognitive tasks (eg, the Wisconsin card sort task) through training, either individually or in a group format, or by placing emphasis on the practice and rehearsal of specific cognitive abilities. So far, cognitive remediation has received more attention in the USA than in Europe [19–21].

Although there is a clear rationale behind cognitive remediation, and comprehensive programmes have been documented (eg, integrated psychological therapy [IPT]) [22], the evidence for its efficacy has been mixed [18]. While most studies are effective in improving specific cognitive deficits within the experimental context, there is less evidence for generalization to other cognitive skills or to the patient's social and occupational functioning. Hogarty and Flesher [23] have argued that the cognitive deficits found in schizophrenia are too severe and pervasive to allow any significant benefits from cognitive rehabilitation. However, Wykes *et al* [24] have shown, in a small randomized controlled trial (RCT) focusing on executive functioning deficits, that therapy implemented on an individualized rather than a standardized group basis improved self-esteem and cognitive deficits. Furthermore, although there were no consistent changes in symptoms or social functioning between the groups, social functioning improved at outcome when a particular threshold was reached. Spaulding *et al* [25] also reported that intensive cognitive rehabilitative treatment had benefits in social competence, as measured by their patients' response to videotaped vignettes. Although these data are promising, the individualized and intensive approach required for any improvements to be manifest has hindered the incorporation of cognitive remediation into standard clinical practice.

Occupational therapy

There is a well-known relationship between engagement in meaningful occupation and health status in both the general population [26] and individuals with mental health problems [27]. The beneficial effects of meaningful occupation lie in structuring time, increasing self-esteem and self-image, developing goals and social relationships, providing a sense of relationship with society, and defining social status. The importance attached to meaningful daytime activities is reinforced by the findings from surveys of patients' priorities with regard to service provision, which listed housing and employment as patients' most urgent priorities.

Occupational therapy tends to occur routinely on inpatient wards, and seems to be valued by those who engage in it [28]. However, specific programmes for vocational rehabilitation — including sheltered workshops, transitional employment programmes, job clubs and supported employment programmes, placement, and 'job coach' models — have been more mixed in their success [29]. Unfortunately, most of the evidence consists of uncontrolled descriptive studies with time-limited interventions and short-term follow up, while the benefits may only become apparent in the long term. For example, Leff *et al* [30] showed that work-related activity made to change in mental state after one-year follow up but showed a significant alteration after five-year follow up, with participants reporting increased freedom and autonomy and enhanced social networks.

Bond *et al* [31] reviewed 13 studies of vocational rehabilitation programmes and concluded that supported employment models were significantly more effective in achieving successful placements in competitive employment compared with conventional approaches. Successful programmes tend to be flexible, integrate clinical and vocational support (rather than occurring in isolation), and cover a range of work opportunities catering for different levels of needs to avoid either overstimulation or understimulation of patients. The 'place-and-train' model seems much more effective than the more traditional 'train-and-place' approach, with patients being able to earn extra money rather than remaining on unpaid training courses. Most importantly, programmes need to take into consideration patients' preferences, reflecting the principles of normalization rather than the rigid prescription of services. This has led to the recent shift away from traditional sheltered workshops and toward supported placement models, and is due to the poor image and stigma associated with sheltered workshops and the importance of 'valued social position' to patients' self-esteem [32].

Cognitive-behaviour therapy

It is now fairly well-established that psychodynamic psychotherapy is not efficacious in the treatment of schizophrenia [33]; however, CBT has proved much more promising in this area. The main assumption behind CBT is that the occurrence and maintenance of psychological difficulties is mediated by cognitive (the way people think or interpret events) and behavioural (what people do and how they feel in response to events) factors [34]. Therapy aims to break the vicious circle between thoughts, feelings and behaviours by helping people to learn more adaptive ways of thinking and coping, which then leads to reduction in distress.

Psychological interventions with specific symptoms

The recent emphasis in studying and generating psychological models of individual symptoms [35], rather than targeting the broad syndrome of schizophrenia, has paved the way for the development of psychological interventions for psychotic symptoms. This body of work has concentrated on the two most common positive symptoms (ie, delusions and hallucinations).

Hallucinations

Treatment of hallucinations has so far concentrated on auditory hallucinations: visual, olfactory and tactile hallucinations have received little attention. This results from the considerable interest in psychological models of auditory hallucinations. Although there is no agreed consensus on the origin of voices, most assume that they are associated with dysfunctional speech processing in some way. It has also been observed that hallucinations are worse under conditions of increased arousal [36], and that the beliefs and attributions patients have about the voices mediate levels of distress [37]. These models suggest that the following strategies may be effective: (i) some form of compensatory coping for dealing with the underlying deficits; (ii) reducing arousal; and (iii) modifying beliefs about the hallucinatory experiences.

The types of intervention differ in emphasis on behavioural and/or cognitive techniques (*see* Table 5.2) and on the psychological model that they are based on. Different measures of outcome are used in different studies, reflecting the multidimensionality of hallucinations. For example, in addition to the frequency and intensity of voices, variables (eg, level of distress, perceived control, preoccupation, and compliance with voices) are dimensions that may vary independently of each other over the course of therapy.

Many of the studies in the literature are uncontrolled case studies and therefore results need to be interpreted with due caution; more recent studies have benefited from improved methodology. In a small study using a 'focusing/re-attribution' intervention, Bentall *et al* [38] found that three out of six patients re-attributed the voices to themselves. A further three patients reported a reduced duration of hallucinations and of distress associated with them, with a modest degree of change. Haddock *et al* [39] reported on a comparison between 'distraction' and 'focusing' approaches in a small RCT. They found that both strategies were effective in significantly reducing the amount of time that the patient spent hallucinating and the level disruption that the voices caused; however, there was a trend for the 'focusing' intervention to significantly increase self-esteem, whereas the 'distraction' approach tended to decrease self-esteem. In an uncontrolled study, Nelson *et al* [40] also found that distraction techniques, such as listening to music using a personal stereo, were limited due to their failure to generalize outside of the period when the stereo is in use. It is becoming increasingly clear that helping the patient to both expose themselves to the content of the voices, in order to reduce the anxiety surrounding them [41], and examine people's beliefs about their voices [37] are more useful strategies than distraction, and, in addition, is more acceptable to 'voice-hearers' [42]. In a small series of case-studies, Chadwick and Birchwood [37] showed that patients' distress and voice-driven behaviour were shaped by their beliefs about the voices' power, identity and knowledge. Challenging these beliefs verbally and with empirical testing led to a reduction in the strength of beliefs in three out of four cases, with the degree of conviction falling from close to 100% to less than 25% for most beliefs.

Types of treatment reported for auditory hallucinations		
Type of approach	**Intervention**	**Content of therapy**
Compensation	Distraction	Attentional resources are redirected through the introduction of competing stimuli (eg, use of personal stereos, doing activities, reading or speaking out loud). Activities using muscles associated with subvocalization tend to be the most successful. Emphasis should be given to the use of techniques that are easily integrated in normal daily life
	Monaural occlusion	Wearing an earplug (either left or right ear)
	Thought stopping	Patient shouts, "Stop it!" (either out loud or internally), when hallucinations occur; snapping of an elastic band against the wrist can also be successful
	Coping skills enhancement (CSE) [43]	Identifies and refines patients' own effective naturally occurring coping strategies; classified as cognitive (eg, self instruction), behavioural (eg, increasing activity levels), modification of sensory input (eg, wearing headphones), modification of physiological state (eg, relaxation)
Anxiety reduction	Anxiety management	Relaxation and breathing techniques aimed at reducing general levels of anxiety
	Systematic desensitization	Desensitization of antecedent and/or concurrent phenomena associated with occurrence or worsening of hallucinations
	Self monitoring	Self monitoring (eg, use of diaries) of the form, frequency, situations and feelings associated with voices. Has to be done concurrently rather than retrospectively. Monitoring may help to increase perceived control at the same time as serving as exposure. Should also be used as a baseline assessment tool before implementing other interventions
	Controlled exposure	If possible, teaching and helping patients to elicit and dismiss their voices, therefore increasing sense of control
Cognitive	Focusing	Gradual exposure to the content of hallucinations, discussion of meaning and beliefs surrounding them, leading to recognition that voices are internally generated
	Belief modification [44]	Based on Chadwick's ABC model (A = Activating event [ie, the voice]; B = Beliefs about the voice; and C = Consequences [both emotional and behavioural]), where beliefs mediate the link between voices and distress experienced. Beliefs tend to revolve around the themes of identity (benevolent versus malevolent), power (over patient and/or other people), control (over voice and compliance), and knowledge (of the patient) of voices. Therapy concentrates on changing target beliefs about omnipotence, malevolence and compliance, rather than actual occurrence

Table 5.2.

It is now becoming recognised that medication-resistant hallucinations are also extremely difficult to reduce using psychological means. However, an increase in perceived control over the hallucinations or a reduction in associated distress may have an enormous effect on quality of life even if the frequency of the hallucinations has not changed. Therefore, it is possible to make a significant impact on patients' lives by changing associated factors such as distress, controllability or beliefs about the voices. In addition, recent studies suggest that the group therapy format may be advantageous in helping people cope with their hallucinations [45,46].

Delusions

Again, there is no consensus model to explain the formation and maintenance of delusions, although most clinicians agree that delusions share many characteristics with normal beliefs (eg, resistance to change and a bias for confirmatory evidence). Current models of delusions emphasise the importance of unusual experiences in driving delusional explanations, presence of reasoning biases (eg, a 'jump-to-conclusions' reasoning style), motivational aspects of delusions in defending against underlying poor self-esteem, and the impact of a 'theory of mind' deficit in forming beliefs about the self and others in a social universe [47].

Delusions are multidimensional in a similar manner to hallucinations. Different dimensions (eg, levels of conviction, preoccupation, interference, accommodation, and distress) can vary independently over the course of therapy [48]. Although fewer studies have investigated CBT approaches to delusions, such studies tend to be better controlled and have a larger number of participants [49,50]. The types of tech-

Psychological interventions with delusions	
Intervention	Techniques
Belief modification	Delusions are organised in a hierarchy, with least strongly held beliefs being tackled first. The delusions themselves are not challenged immediately, but rather the evidence supporting them is examined and the distress is targeted. Confrontation is minimized to avoid psychological reactance
Reality testing	Behavioural experiments are set up to test out the reality of the delusions and their supporting evidence. These should be carried out in concert with structured verbal challenge
Attribution therapy	Based on the finding that paranoid patients tend to blame other people rather than the situation for everyday negative events [51]. Re attributing meaningful events to situational rather than personal causes

Table 5.3.

niques used for delusional modification include reality testing [49,50,52] and, more recently, attribution therapy (ie, re-attributing meaningful events to situational rather than personal causes [*see* Table 5.3]) [51]. Overall, it is becoming apparent that delusions are more easily modified by psychological means than hallucinations.

Cognitive-behaviour therapy packages

General CBT packages have now been developed for a range of psychotic patients, from early-onset to drug-resistant patients with chronic schizophrenia, and have been adapted from the widespread application of CBT in neurotic disorders [34]. The emphasis is on management rather than treatment of the psychotic illness, although significant reductions in the occurrence of delusions can be obtained. Therapy is recommended to last between six and 12 months. All packages tend to be based on an individualized formulation approach that takes into account the heterogeneity of symptoms found in psychosis, the continuum of severity of symptoms, and the plethora of emotional secondary disturbances experienced by psychotic patients. It is crucial that individuals are able to engage in the therapy (ie, that the individual patient is able to create and sustain a therapeutic relationship and rapport with the therapist [*see* Table 5.4]).

There have been a number of RCTs published in the UK [53–59], and the largest study to date (SOCRATES — Study of Cognitive Reality Alignment Therapy in Early Schizophrenia) is reaching its final stages. However, there are a number of treatment manuals currently available [44,60,61].

Cognitive behaviour therapy for psychosis	
Issues in therapy	Coping with disability Management of psychotic symptoms Management of emotional problems Addressing interpersonal/intrapsychic issues
Techniques used in therapy	Didactic psychoeducation Normalization and reframing of psychotic symptoms Problem solving Behavioural techniques Cognitive techniques Schema focused techniques Supportive counselling
Stages of therapy	Engagement and assessment Promoting self regulation of psychotic symptoms (coping) Developing shared formulation of psychosis Addressing delusions and beliefs about voices Addressing dysfunctional assumptions about self and others Addressing social disability and risk of relapse

Table 5.4. Adapted with permission from [61].

Kuipers *et al* [57] reported a 25% reduction in symptom scores, produced mainly by changes in delusions but also to a lesser extent in hallucinations. This is similar to the effects of clozapine on drug-resistant patients found in some studies [62]. However, no significant changes were found in levels of depression or social functioning. Fifty percent of the therapy group were treatment responders. Predictors of good outcome included cognitive flexibility concerning delusions, however, neither intelligence quotient (IQ) nor severity of illness were related to treatment response [63]. This kind of therapy is highly acceptable to patients, with only an 11% drop-out rate (mostly from the control group), and 80% of individuals reporting satisfaction with the treatment received. Furthermore, patients continued to improve even after therapy was terminated, with delusional distress and frequency of hallucinations being further significantly reduced at 18-months follow up [58]. Overall, Kuipers *et al* [57,58] reported that the costs of CBT were offset by reductions in use of services and associated costs during follow up.

In an extended, nonrandomised, pilot study using the 'normalising' approach, Kingdon and Turkington [60] found that 35 out of 65 patients were free of acute psychotic symptoms after five-year follow up. However, there was no comparison group or objective assessment of symptoms. In a more rigorous RCT of this approach, Sensky *et al* [59] found that symptom improvements just failed to reach significance at the end of therapy, but continued improvements gave significant differences at 18-month follow up, these findings supported the Kuipers *et al* study [58].

Most of the CBT packages have been targeted at individuals who are well enough to attend outpatient appointments, but who have distressing residual symptoms. However, in a small RCT, Drury *et al* [64,65] demonstrated that even acute inpatients undergoing a florid psychotic episode may be accessible to psychological intervention. Drury *et al* gave patients in the treatment group the following four individual and group procedures: (i) individual cognitive therapy; (ii) group cognitive therapy; (iii) family engagement; and (iv) structured activity programme away from the ward. The treatment programme took on average eight hours a week over a 12-week period. They found that the treatment group showed a more significantly marked decline in positive symptoms, and a 25–50% reduction in recovery time (depending on the definition used). Furthermore, the impact of treatment extended beyond positive symptoms to include insight, dysphoria and 'low-level' psychotic thinking. At nine-months follow up, 5% of the treatment group (compared with 56% of the control group) showed moderate or severe residual symptoms. Although 35% of their original sample were excluded because the patients involved did not disclose their symptoms, adhere to prescribed medication or refused to engage in the therapy programme. This study, nevertheless, demonstrates that psychological input, even during the acute phase, can have a significant impact on recovery on at least two-thirds of a typical inner-city sample of hospitalized patients with psychosis.

A smaller study compared CBT with supportive counselling for a group of acutely ill patients [66]. The treatment was low intensity: a total of eight-hours duration in the CBT group, and five-hours duration in the counselling group. Both groups showed a reduction in symptom scores during therapy, although the two groups did not differ from each other. At two-year follow up the number of patients who relapsed, the number of relapses and the time to recurrence of psychotic symptoms were lower in the CBT group, however, the time to readmission was shorter. This suggests that even low-intensity, supportive counselling may be beneficial in reducing psychotic symptoms.

Tarrier *et al* have also found that supportive counselling can be beneficial [55]. In a large study comparing Coping Strategy Enhancement (CSE; adapted for other psychotic symptoms as well as for hallucinations) with supportive counselling and standard care, they found that the supportive counselling group was mid-way in outcome between the other two groups, although only the CSE group showed significant differences in symptom severity and number of positive symptoms compared with the standard care group. Overall, patients in the CSE group were eight times more likely than those in the routine care group to have a 50% reduction in positive symptom score. The significant difference between the CSE and the routine care group in severity of positive symptoms remained at a one-year follow-up [56].

Medication compliance

Many patients do not adhere to their medication regimen, and noncompliance incurs substantial individual and social costs in terms of untreated morbidity and relapse. Patients cease taking their medication for a variety of reasons, including intolerance of side effects, lack of insight, fears about stigma or dependency, or the natural tendency to stop taking medication when one feels well. Purely psychoeducational or didactic approaches have limited effectiveness. Medication compliance therapy (or medication adherence) is based on a combination of CBT techniques, and motivational interviewing, which is commonly used in the addictions (*see* Table 5.5) [67]. Compliance therapy has been evaluated by RCT, and has been found to lead to significant improvements in attitudes to medication, insight, and compliance [68]. These advantages were maintained over an 18-month period, and global social functioning and time of survival in the community prior to readmission were increased [69]. The brevity of the therapy (four to six sessions, with possible additional booster sessions) combined with its clinical effectiveness make it relatively cost-effective [70].

Early intervention

A third paradigm of intervention, called 'early intervention' (EI), has been developed by McGorry *et al* at the Early Psychosis Prevention and Intervention Centre (EPPIC), Australia [71]. A number of European centres have since been set up, for example in

51

Compliance therapy	
Phases of therapy	**Content of therapy**
1. Eliciting patient's stance towards medication	Rapport building. Exploring patient's conceptualization of problems. Review illness and medication history Psychoeducation based on normalizing rationale
2. Exploring ambivalence to medication	Discussing patient's misgivings about medication (misconceptions about medication, side effects, stigma, denial of psychological difficulties, natural tendency to stop medication when well). Pros and cons of taking medication examined (homing in on benefits). Psycho education about medication. If appropriate exploring delu sional explanations which pose resistance to adherence
3. Treatment maintenance	Reframing use of medication as free choice. Combating stigma. Discussion of prodromal symptoms. 'Staying well' in context of chronic illness

Table 5.5. Adapted with permission from [68].

Birmingham, UK [72], and Amsterdam, The Netherlands [73]. EI promotes the establishment of services rather than representing a type of therapy *per se*. Unlike the other two paradigms, which concentrate on treatment of distressing symptoms and psychological difficulties and amelioration of social, physical or cognitive disabilities (the rehabilitation model), EI aims to prevent, abort or ameliorate florid relapse during the critical period around the first onset of the illness. Such an approach is deemed to have beneficial long-term repercussions for the following reasons: (i) the duration of untreated psychosis (the 'treatment lag') is linked to the early course of schizophrenia [74]; (ii) the early phase of psychosis and the variables which influence it are thought to be formative, with crucial biological and psychosocial changes being laid down in this critical period [75]; and (iii) each relapse brings with it an increased risk of future relapse and accelerating social disablement.

EI strategies include the following three key elements: (i) early detection of 'at risk' or prodromal mental states; (ii) early treatment of the first psychotic episode; and (iii) interventions targeted during the early phase of psychosis (the 'critical period').

Yung *et al* [76] have shown that it is possible to identify a group particularly vulnerable to impending psychosis using a combination of genetic, personality and prodromal risk factors in a generalized outpatient service for adolescents. They found that 40% of their high-risk group made the transition to psychosis within six months. Early detection paves the way for potential intervention before the onset of psychosis, with the avoidance of hospitalization and the use of low-dose medication being high priorities. Nevertheless, issues of possibly unnecessary or premature labelling, stigma and treatment arise and any decision to treat early should be considered carefully [77].

Pioneering services, such as EPPIC, have been extremely influential in setting up services for first-onset patients in the UK and other parts of Europe, although the impact of EI has yet to be established by RCT and prospective research studies. A naturalistic study of EPPIC found that at least one-third of all patients with first-episode psychosis could be assessed and treated in the community during the acute phase of the illness. Both hospitalized and nonhospitalized individuals could in general be managed by low-dose antipsychotic medication, with 80% responding to treatment and 63% being in remission after three months [78]. Only one study so far has investigated the role of CBT in this group [79]: the CBT group had better outcomes on a scale of integration/sealing over (a measure of patients' adaptation to the illness), but were more depressed. However, this was not a randomized trial, and further research is needed in this area. Although robust evaluations are still lacking in both the efficacy and the effectiveness of early and preventative interventions, the EI movement is starting to succeed in replacing the old Kraepelinian model of psychosis as 'doomed from the womb' with a climate of renewed optimism.

Conclusion

Recent years have seen the development of a plethora of psychosocial interventions. It is now recognised that improving the course of schizophrenia means going beyond simple symptom control, and involves the psychosocial reintegration of patients in their communities. However, different services differ markedly in the degree of implementation of each of the approaches described above, and even the most established successful therapies, for example family interventions, are not yet routinely included in the care plan approach. Radical organisational changes will, therefore, need to be made in future services to accommodate family and psychosocial management approaches for psychosis.

References

1. Hogarty GE, Ulrich RF. **The limitations of antipsychotic medication on schizophrenia relapse and adjustment and the contributions of psychosocial treatment.** *J Psychiatr Res* 1998; **32**:243–250.

2. Nuechterlein KH. **Vullnerability models for schizophrenia: State of the Art.** In: *Search for the Causes of Schizophrenia.* Edited by: WFGH Hafner and W Janzarik. Heidelberg: Springer-Verlag; 1987, 297–316.

3. Fadden G, Bebbington P, Kuipers L. **Caring and its burden.** *Br J Psychiatry* 1987; **151**:660–667.

4. Brown G. **The discovery of Expressed Emotion: induction or deduction.** In: *Expressed Emotion in Families.* Edited by JPLCE Vaughn. New York: Guildford Press; 1985.

5. Bebbington P, Kuipers L. **The predictive utility of Expressed Emotion in schizophrenia: An aggregate analysis.** *Psychol Med* 1994; **24**:707–718.

6. Penn DL, Mueser KT. **Research update on the psychosocial treatment of schizophrenia.** *Am J Psychiatry* 1996; **153**: 607–617.

7. Tarrier N, Barrowclough C. **Family interventions in schizophrenia and their long-term outcomes.** *Int J Ment Health* 1995; **24**(3):38–53.

8. Herzog T. **Nurses, patients and relatives: A study of family patterns on psychiatric wards.** In: *Family Intervention in Schizophrenia: Experiences and Orientations in Europe.* Edited by CLCG. Milan: Invernizzi. ARS; 1992.

9. Moore E, Ball R, Kuipers L. **Expressed Emotion in staff working with the long-term adult mentally ill.** *Br J Psychiatry* 1992; **161**:802–808.

10. Tarrier N, Lowson K, Barrowclough C. **Some aspects of family interventions in schizophrenia. II: Financial considerations.** *Br J Psychiatry* 1991; **159**:481–484.

11. Liberman RP, Mueser KT, Wallace CG. **Social skills training for schizophrenic individuals at risk for relapse.** *Am J Psychiatry* 1986; **143**:523–526.

12. Wirshing WC, Marder SR, Eckman T *et al.* **Acquisition and retention of skills training methods in chronic schizophrenic outpatients.** *Psychopharmacol Bull* 1992; **28**:241–245.

13. Marder SR, Wirshing WC, Mintz J *et al.* **Two-year outcome of social skills, training and group psychotherapy for outpatients with schizophrenia.** *Am J Psychiatry* 1996; **153**:1585–1592.

14. Benton MK, Schroeder HE. **Social skills training with schizophrenics: a meta-analytic evaluation.** *J Consult Clin Psychol* 1990; **58**:741–747.

15. Wykes T, Dunn G. **Cognitive deficit and the prediction of rehabilitation success in a chronic psychiatric group.** *Psychol Med* 1992; **22**:389-398.

16. Spaulding WD, Fleming, SK, Reed D *et al.* **Cognitive functioning in schizophrenia: Implications for psychiatric rehabilitation.** *Schizophr Bull* 1999; **25**:275-289.

17. Mueser KT, Bellack A, Douglas MS *et al.* **Prediction of social skills acquisition in schizophrenic and major affective disorder patients from memory and symptomatology.** *Psychiatry Res* 1991; **37**:281-296.

18. Bellack AS, Gold JM, Buchanan RW. **Cognitive rehabilitation for schizophrenia: Problems, prospects and strategies.** *Schizophr Bull* 1999; **25**:257-274.

19. Hogarty GE, Flesher S. **Developmental theory for a cognitive enhancement therapy of schizophrenia.** *Schizophr Bull* 1999; **25**:677–692.

20. Hogarty GE, Flesher S. **Cognitive remediation in schizophrenia: proceed... with caution.** *Schizophr Bull* 1992; 18:51–57.

21. Spring BJ, Ravdin L. **Cognitive remediation in schizophrenia: should we attempt it?** *Schizophr Bull* 1992; **18**:15–20.

22. Brenner H, Roder V, Hodel B *et al. Integrated Psychological Therapy for Schizophrenia Patients.* Toronto: Hogrefe & Huber; 1994.

23. Hogarty GE, Flesher S. **Cognitive remediation in schizophrenia: proceed... with caution!** *Schizophr Bull* 1992; **18**:51–57.

24. Wykes T, Reeder C, Corner J *et al.* **The effects of neurocognitive remediation on executive processing in patients with schizophrenia.** *Schizophr Bull* 1999; **25**:291-309.

25. Spaulding WD, Reed D, Storzbach D *et al.* **The effects of a remediational approach to cognitive therapy for schizophrenia.** In: *Outcome and Innovation in Psychological Treatment of Schizophrenia.* Edited by T Wykes, N Tarrier and S Lewis. London: John Wiley & Sons; 1998.

26. Warr P. *Work, Unemployment and mental Health.* Oxford: Oxford University Press; 1987.

27. Warner R. *Recovery from Schizophrenia.* London: Routledge; 1985.

28. Chadwick PK. *Schizophrenia: The Positive Perspective.* London, Routledge; 1997.

29. Harding CM, Strauss JS, Hafez H *et al. Work and mental illness: Towards an integration of treatment and rehabilitation.* In: **Schizophrenia: Breaking Down the Barriers.** Edited by SG Holliday, RJ Ancill and GW McEwan. Chichester: John Wiley & Sons, Inc.; 1996, 39–61.

30. Leff J, Thornicroft G, Coxhead N *et al.* **The TAPS Project. 22: A five-year follow-up of long-stay psychiatric patients discharged to the community.** *Br J Psychiatry Suppl* 1994; **25**:13–17.

31. Bond GR, Drake RE, Mueser KT *et al.* **An update on supported employment for people with severe mental illness.** *Psychiatr Serv* 1997; **48**:335–346.

32. Dick N, Shepherd G. **Work and mental health: A preliminary test of Warr's model in sheltered workshops for the mentally ill.** *J Ment Health* 1994; **3**:387–400.

33. Gunderson JG, Frank AF, Katz HM *et al.* **Effects of psychotherapy in schizophrenia: II. Comparative outcome of two forms of treatment.** *Schizophr Bull* 1984; **10**:564–598.

34. Beck AT, Rush AJ, Shaw BF *et al. Cognitive Therapy of Depression.* New York: Guildford Press; 1979.

35. Bentall RP. *Reconstructing Schizophrenia*. London: Routledge; 1990.

36. Margo A, Hemsley DR, Slade PD. **The effects of varying auditory input on schizophrenic hallucinations.** *Br J Psychiatry* 1981; **139**:122–127.

37. Chadwick P, Birchwood M. **The omnipotence of voices. A cognitive approach to auditory hallucinations.** *Br J Psychiatry* 1994; **164**:190–201.

38. Bentall RP, Haddock G, Slade PD. **Cognitive behaviour therapy for persistent auditory hallucinations: From theory to therapy.** *Behaviour Therapy* 1994; **25**:51–66.

39. Haddock G, Bentall RP, Slade PD. **Psychological treatment of auditory hallucinations: Focusing or distraction?** In: *Cognitive-behavioural Interventions with Psychotic Disorders*. Edited by G Haddock and P Slade. London: Routledge; 1996.

40. Nelson HE, Thrasher S, Barnes TRE. **Practical ways of alleviating auditory hallucinations.** *Br Med J* 1991; **302**:307.

41. Persaud R, Marks I. **A pilot study of exposure and control of chronic auditory hallucinations.** *Br J Psychiatry* 1995; **167**:45-50.

42. Romme MA, Escher AD. *Accepting Voices*. London: Mind Publications; 1994.

43. Tarrier N, Harwood S, Yusupoff L *et al.* **Coping Strategy Enhancement (CSE): A method of treating residual schizophrenic symptoms.** *Behav Psychother* 1990; **18**:283–293.

44. Chadwick PDJ, Birchwood M, Trower P. *Cognitive Therapy with Delusions and Voices*. Chichester: John Wiley & Sons, Inc.; 1996.

45. Wykes T, Parr AM, Landau S. **Group CBT for auditory hallucinations. Exploratory study of effectiveness.** *Br J Psychiatry* 1999; **175**:180–185.

46. Chadwick PDJ *et al.* **Group CBT for auditory hallucinations.** *Behaviour, Res Therapy* 2000(in press).

47. Garety PA, Freeman D. **Cognitive approaches to delusions: A critical review of theories and evidence.** *Br J Clin Psychol* 1999; **38**(pt. 2):113–154.

48. Brett-Jones J, Garety PA, Hemsley DR. **Measuring delusional experiences: A method and its application.** *Br J Clin Psychol* 1987; **26**:257–265.

49. Chadwick PD, Lowe CF. **Measurement and modification of delusional beliefs.** *J Consult Clin Psychol* 1990; **58**:225–232.

50. Chadwick PD, Lowe CF. **A cognitive approach to measuring and modifying delusions.** *Behav Res Ther* 1994; **32**:355–367.

51. Kinderman P, Bentall RP. **Causal attributions in paranoia and depression: Internal, personal and situational attributions for negative events.** *J Abnorm Psychol* 1997; **106**:341–345.

52. Lowe CF, Chadwick PDJ. **Verbal control of delusions.** *Behaviour Therapy* 1990; **21**:461–479.

53. Tarrier N, Beckett R, Harwood S *et al.* **A trial of two cognitive-behavioural methods of treating drug-resistant residual psychotic symptoms in schizophrenic patients: I: Outcome.** *Br J Psychiatry* 1993; **162**:524–532.

54. Tarrier N, Sharpe L, Beckett R *et al.* **A trial of two cognitive-behavioural methods of treating drug-resistant residual psychotic symptoms in schizophrenic patients: II: Treatment-specific changes in coping and problem-solving skills.** *Social Psychiatry Psychiatr Epidemiol* 1993; **28**:5–10.

55. Tarrier N, Yusupoff L, Kinney C *et al.* **Randomised controlled trial of intensive cognitive behaviour therapy for patients with chronic schizophrenia.** *Br Med J* 1998; **317**:303–307.

56. Tarrier N, Wittkowski A, Kinney C *et al.* **The durability of the effects of cognitive-behaviour therapy in the treatment of chronic schizophrenia: Twelve months follow-up.** *Br J Psychiatry* 1999; **174**:500–504.

57. Kuipers E, Garety PA, Fowler D *et al.* **London–East Anglia randomised controlled trial of cognitive-behavioural therapy for psychosis. I: Effects of treatment phase.** *Br J Psychiatry* 1997; **171**:319–327.

58. Kuipers E, Fowler D, Garety PA *et al.* **London–East Anglia randomised controlled trial of cognitive-behavioural therapy for psychosis. III: Follow-up and economic evaluation at 18 months.** *Br J Psychiatry* 1998; **173**:61–68.

59. Sensky T, Turkington D, Kingdon D *et al.* **A randomised controlled trial of cognitive-behavioral therapy for persistent symptoms in schizophrenia resistant to medication.** *Arch Gen Psychiatry* 2000; **57**:165–172.

60. Kingdon DG, Turkington D. *Cognitive–Behavioural Therapy of Schizophrenia.* Erlbaum; 1994.

61. Fowler D, Garety PA, Kuipers E. *Cognitive–Behaviour Therapy for Psychosis.* Chichester: John Wiley & Sons, Inc.; 1995.

62. Kane JM, Honingfeld G, Singer J *et al.* **Clozapine for the treatment-resistant schizophrenic: A double blind comparison with chlorpromazine.** *Arch Gen Psychiatry* 1988; **45**:789–796.

63. Garety PA, Fowler D, Kuipers E *et al.* **London–East Anglia randomised controlled trial of cognitive-behavioural therapy for psychosis. II: Predictors of outcome.** *Br J Psychiatry* 1997; **171**:420–426.

64. Drury V, Birchwood M, Cochrane R *et al.* **Cognitive therapy and recovery from acute psychosis: A controlled trial. I: Impact on psychotic symptoms.** *Br J Psychiatry* 1996; **169**:593–601.

65. Drury V, Birchwood M, Cochrane R *et al.* **Cognitive therapy and recovery from acute psychosis: A controlled trial. II: Impact on recovery time.** *Br J Psychiatry* 1996; **169**:602–607.

66. Haddock G, Tarrier N, Morrison AP *et al.* **A pilot study evaluating the effectiveness of individual inpatient cognitive-behavioural therapy in early psychosis.** *Social Psychiatr Psychiatric Epidemiol* 1999; **34**:254–258.

67. Rollnick S, Heather N, Bell A. **Negotiating behaviour change in medical settings: The development of a brief motivational interviewing.** *J Ment Health* 1992; **1**:25–37.

68. Kemp R, David A, Hayward P. **Compliance therapy: An intervention targeting insight and treatment adherence in psychotic patients.** *Behav Cognitive Psychother* 1996; **24**:331–350.

69. Kemp R, Kirov G, Everitt B *et al.* **Randomised controlled trial of compliance therapy: 18 months follow-up.** *Br J Psychiatry* 1998; **172**:413–419.

70. Healey A, Knapp M, Astin J *et al.* **Cost-effectiveness evaluation of compliance therapy for people with psychosis.** *Br J Psychiatry* 1998; **172**:420–424.

71. McGorry PD, Edwards J, Mihalopoulos C *et al.* **Early Psychosis Prevention and Intervention Centre (EPPIC): An evolving system of early detection and optimal management.** *Schizophr Bull* 1996; **22**:305–326.

72. Birchwood M, McGorry P, Jackson H. **Early intervention in schizophrenia.** *Br J Psychiatry* 1997; **170**:2–5.

73. Linszen D, Lenior M, de Haan L *et al.* **Early intervention, untreated psychosis and the course of early schizophrenia.** *Br J Psychiatry* 1998; **172**(suppl. 33):84-89.

74. Loebel AD, Liberman JA, Alvir JM *et al.* **Duration of psychosis and outcome in first episode schizophrenia.** *Am J Psychiatry* 1992; **149**:1183–1188.

75. Birchwood M, Todd P, Jackson C. **Early intervention in psychosis: The critical period hypothesis.** *Br J Psychiatry* 1998; **172**(suppl. 33):53–59.

76. Yung AR, Phillips L, McGorry PD *et al.* **Prediction of psychosis.** *Br J Psychiatry* 1998; **172**(suppl. 33):14–20.

77. Yung AR, McGorry PD. **Is pre-psychotic intervention realistic in schizophrenia and related disorders?** *Australian New Zealand J Psychiatry* 1997; **31**:799–805.

78. Power P, Elkins K, Adlard S *et al.* **Analysis of the initial treatment phase in first-episode psychosis.** *Br J Psychiatry* 1998; **172**(suppl. 33):71–76.

79. Jackson H, McGorry P, Edwards J *et al.* **Cognitively-oriented psychotherapy for early psychosis (COPE): Preliminary results.** *Br J Psychiatry* 1998; **172**(suppl. 33):93–100.